KU-286-087

369 0246782

JOHN KILLICK was a teacher for 30 years, and has been a writer all his life. He has published books of his own po......... ....orking with......................... .....he'd a number of po......n nurs...h.m......pr.de, libraries and arts centr... With Kate All.n, Joh.n crea.ed and moderates the website www.dementiapositive.co.uk. He as edited six books of poems by people with dementia, and co-authored books on communication and on creativity. He has written many articles and book chapters, and given many workshops in the UK and abroad. He has also made a number of appearances on radio and TV.

MONKLANDS HOSPITAL
LIBRARY
MONKSCOURT AVENUE
AIRDRIE ML60'S
☎0123671200

By the same author:

Playfulness and Dementia: A Practical Guide
(Jessica Kingsley, 2012)

*Creativity and Communication in Persons with Dementia:
A Practical Guide* (with Claire Craig, Jessica Kingsley, 2011)

Communication and the Care of People with Dementia
(with Kate Allan, Open University Press, 2001)

DEMENTIA POSITIVE

A HANDBOOK BASED ON LIVED EXPERIENCES

For everyone wishing to improve the lives
of those with dementia

JOHN KILLICK

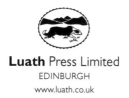

Luath Press Limited
EDINBURGH
www.luath.co.uk

BARCODE NO: 36902460782
CLASS NO: WT 155 KIL
PRICE: 9.99
DATE: 23/10/13

First published 2013

ISBN: 978-1-908373-57-1

The paper used in this book is recyclable. It is made from
low chlorine pulps produced in a low energy, low emission
manner from renewable forests.

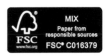

Printed and bound by
The Charlesworth Group, Wakefield

Typeset in 10.5 point Sabon and Gill
by 3btype.com

The author's right to be identified as author of this
work under the Copyright, Designs and Patents Act 1988
has been asserted.

© John Killick

MONKLANDS HOSPITAL
LIBRARY
MONKSCOURT AVENUE
AIRDRIE ML60JS
01236712005

You did then what you knew how to do and when you
knew better you did better.

MAYA ANGELOU

We receive and we lose, and we must try to achieve
gratitude; and with that gratitude to embrace with whole
hearts whatever of life that remains after the losses.

ANDRE DUBUS

I dwell in Possibility   EMILY DICKINSON

CONTENTS

ACKNOWLEDGEMENTS

I would especially like to express my gratitude to Caroline Brown, Kate Grillet and Helen Finch for their contributions, and for their comments on the manuscript generally. The extracts by all three of these individuals have been specially offered to me for this book. Kate Allan has once again been my sternest, and therefore most valuable, critic. I owe the format of the book to her as well, which I have borrowed from her groundbreaking training resource *Finding Your Way*, alas no longer available. I am also grateful to Cathy Greenblat for the use of one of her wonderful photographs on the cover: this surely sets the tone for what this book is about.

You will already have read three quotations which I have chosen because, despite the fact that dementia was probably not in the writers' minds when they wrote them, I believe they carry the message of this book.

I would like to apply these not just to dementia but specifically to those of us in a supporting role. They are a call to arms, but of the compassionate rather than the military sort. They offer us what I would like to call 'a manageable challenge'.

It's a challenge I took on over twenty years ago, and it's a never-ending one. I have gradually come to see more and more people engaging with a vision of how life with the condition could be, and can be. In this book I want to reflect that vision and their experience.

For myself, I was a teacher for thirty years, and a writer in my spare time. Then I left the classroom behind to live a life in a writer's study. Only that's not how it worked out. I had to earn a living, so I began to take writers' residencies, placements in the community where one can be of use in a different way from writing poems and stories of one's own. I worked first in a women's prison, then a hospice, and latterly in care homes. I began with the life stories of older residents, then I met my first person with dementia.

I knew then that I had found the area I wanted to concentrate on. There was a crying need (sometimes literally) for people's voices to be heard, and written down, and shared back with them. It was a way of confirming for them that they were still there. It was a way of reassuring them that their words were still of importance.

I thought a lot about the process I was engaged in, and I began to listen to what others were saying about the condition, particularly those who had experience of it through family and friends. I realised that there was something about the subject that makes communication and relationships especially important, and wanted to share my viewpoint with others. I believe it has all been leading up to this book.

I can't tell you much about plaques, tangles or drugs – I'm not qualified to do so. I don't deal with diet or exercise – though these are positive strategies which complement those I concentrate on.

My conviction is that one person's experience, however extensive, is by no means the whole story. So eighteen of the nineteen chapters include a section solely dedicated to the words of people with dementia themselves, and those who come into contact with them – family and friends mainly, but some professionals as well, where I thought their insights might be helpful. You can find out where these quotes come from at the back of the book.

In Chapter One I consider the language we use to talk about dementia. It is very important to get the words right. I have decided to use the term 'dementia' sparingly because it becomes monotonous, so when I refer to someone with dementia I often use the word 'person', and sometimes the phrase 'person with the condition'. I also want to avoid the word 'carer' as much as possible, because it always puts the person with dementia into a dependent role. I have decided to use the term 'supporters' for those closest to the person (often referred to in other books as 'primary carers') as well as the rest of family and friends. I am excluding professional carers here: their relationship is necessarily on a different basis. That is not to say that some of what I and others have to say in these pages may not resonate with them, but they are not the main audience I am addressing.

I say I have a vision of how things could be – that's true, but I don't want to stray too far from things as they are. However, there is still so much negativity swirling around this subject, I have no intention of adding to that. I have looked for the upbeat wherever I can find it and it seems justified.

But I don't want you to come away from this introduction with the feeling that I am going to give you lots of dogmatic pieces of advice. I have learnt enough to know that that would be deceiving. We are dealing with, on the one hand, possibly the most complex condition humans can face, and on the other, individuals in all their diversity. So this is a book of hints and potentials, not certainties. If you find me overstepping the mark, please give me a mental wrap on the knuckles!

We have a long way to go in creating the ideal dementia

world. Maybe that is a world in which it never occurs to us to use the word. But starting from where we are now I believe we can all make a difference, however small, in the spirit of the quotations at the head of the book. The first thing we need to do is to stop 'fighting' the condition, as some experts and organizations would have us do, and adopt a mindset of cooperating with it. (I do not mean by this that we should refrain from fighting for the services we believe we deserve!) I am referring to an attitude of acceptance rather than conflict in how dementia is viewed by both person and supporter. That should take us a lot further. I hope to show you some ways in which this can be achieved.

CHAPTER ONE

Talking The Talk

Part One

Some time ago I saw a video about group homes for people in Japan. The strongest message about the kind of support developed there was that those with dementia and those who look after them form a partnership. It was said that they are like a family, exploring relationships and sharing achievements.

The film was made for the Japanese market but I saw the English language version. In this the residents were referred to as 'occupants' and 'cohabitants' and the carers as 'staff members' and 'professionals'. Despite the positive messages contained in the film I felt that the use of these terms undermined its spirit. It made me think anew about the significance of the words we use.

The language in which we talk about any subject is crucial. It reflects our attitudes and beliefs as well as our knowledge and understanding. But that's not all: it can impose narrow limits on our potential for taking on new ideas and ways of acting in the future. In this way language can hold us back from essential learning and growing. It can reinforce our prejudices and confine us within our limitations.

I believe our current ways of talking about dementia often let us down in these ways. If we don't get the words right in talking and thinking about the subject we will never achieve a helpful and realistic understanding of a really complex condition. And this can act like a computer virus spreading throughout the system and infecting all our attempts to get things right in our relationships with people.

Firstly, in the world of professional care it is my view that 'manage' is a weasel word. People are there to be 'managed', and this leads staff into the unthinking adoption of practices which actually work against the person and lead to their disempowerment. As supporters we shouldn't fall into this trap.

Then there is the word 'sufferer'. Whilst it is clear that in certain respects people with dementia do suffer, referring to them as 'sufferers' is objectionable because it puts the condition first, as if the individual's very identity has been subsumed by it. And this means getting rid of the word 'victim' too. It carries similar and even more negative suggestions. The idea that someone may have been targeted in some way is far too simplistic. As for the term 'patient', this carries associations of doctors and hospitals and leaves society's role completely out of the frame. We don't use this term for someone diagnosed with diabetes living in their own home, so why someone with dementia in a similar situation?

I suggest we use the idea of dementia as a disability, with all that that implies of coming to terms and social attitudes, rather than considering it solely as a medical condition, with the emphasis on treatment. This will get around the idea that all the problems a person faces are caused by the state of their brain. I am suspicious of the use of the terms 'illness' and 'disease' in talking about dementia and prefer the word 'condition' which is less specific and more commensurate with the present state of our knowledge.

Looming above all of us is, of course, the term 'Alzheimer's'. Let's trace how this word came to be used and acquire its current associations. What follows is a very brief summary of the views of the English psychologists Mike Bender and Rik Cheston, supplemented by those of the American neurologist Peter Whitehouse.

Over 100 years ago, Dr Alois Alzheimer met Frau Auguste D and attempted to find an explanation for the unusual ways in which she appeared to him. He came under the influence of a celebrated psychiatrist who decided on the basis of this one instance to call it 'Alzheimer's' and include it in a new edition of the textbook he was compiling.

There it lay, innocently undisturbed, until the 1970s, when various organizations were created, national and international. To give them a catchy title in order to attract research funding, the word was promoted. Thus a disease was born.

Since then the drugs companies have proclaimed it and profited hugely. It has been convenient to them to present a worst-case scenario because it attracts cash from scared individuals like you and me. I'm not saying that it's all a con-trick – there is undoubtedly something there to be addressed, but we are dealing here with hype on a large scale, and this seriously interferes with our ability (individually and as a society) to get the thing into some sort of perspective.

As I hope to explain in the next chapter, dementia is a condition which is uniquely responsive to how we regard it and the person labelled with it, so it is unhelpful to all concerned to maintain a negative attitude.

If we ceased using the term 'Alzheimer's' and substituted 'dementia' we wouldn't be much better off. This is because, despite the fact that the latter includes the former and therefore they are not synonymous, they have come to be used as such, and so all the alarming associations have rubbed off on the latter term. In any case a word which means 'without mind' is hardly reassuring, and certainly no more accurate. Really we need to get rid of both terms.

Have we any alternatives? I have scoured the experts for suggestions but without much success. In America the term 'major neurocognitive disorder' is under consideration. In the UK Julian Hughes, a psychiatrist, favours 'acquired diffuse neurocognitive dysfunction', which is probably more accurate but hardly trips off the tongue! We badly need a word (no more than three syllables?) that does the job without carrying the stigma. Any ideas?

Part Two *Other Voices*

Here is someone speaking on an Alzheimer's Society video:

Names have power, like the word 'Alzheimer's'; it terrorises us; it has power over us. When we are prepared to discuss it aloud we might have power over it. There should be no shame in having it, yet people still feel ashamed and people don't talk about it.

And here is Richard Taylor, an American psychologist who has been diagnosed with Alzheimer's Disease, in an extract from a book he has written:

Some words are so powerful because the territory we believe it describes is so scary, is so scandalous, is so sinful, is so gross that we believe if we do not use the word, then we won't think about the territory. In these cases, we have already located the symbol (the word) and the territory (its meaning). We think we can control our fear of the territory by controlling the saying of the word...

Please, sit down with each other and talk first about the territory. Nothing is to be gained, and much will be lost, if saying the words aloud so traumatizes those involved that they do not hear what follows the words *Alzheimer's disease*.

Christine Bryden is a woman with the condition in Australia, and has this warning to offer:

Please don't call us 'dementing' – we are still people separate from our disease, we just have a disease of the brain. If I had cancer you would not refer to me as 'cancerous' would you?

Bob Fay, who has Pick's Disease says:

What a very unfriendly word 'dementia' is. Technically I must have been 'dementing' for about ten years. To me the term suggests insanity – and the dictionaries agree. To be demented implies being frantic, overactive, out of one's mind. I haven't settled on a better term, but I usually say I have Pick's disease or that I have a degenerative brain disease. Sometimes I call myself 'an old Dementonian' but then people think I'm claiming to have had an elitist education!

I shall end this section with the words of Joanne Koenig Coste, a supporter who has realised the power of words to distort and obstruct:

Let's try some new vocabulary here, some reframing:

Instead of 'wandering'	how about 'sightseeing'?
for 'incontinence'	'unplanned leakage'
'aggressive'	'lets her needs be known'
'rummaging'	'good bargain basement technique'
'agitated'	'spirited'
'hoarding'	'a collection of favourite things'
for 'dementia'	'no worries for tomorrow'

End Note

I hope I have convinced you that the words we use to describe or refer to something are important. They are a give-away as to our attitude. So in order to think sensibly about this subject we need to watch our language and the language of other people very carefully, not least that very word 'dementia' which is on the cover of this book. In conjunction with the word 'positive' it really reads like a contradiction in terms. I will never forget the words of Ian McQueen:

> Every time someone uses the word I think they are saying 'Give him another kick!'

CHAPTER TWO **What Kind of Thing is Dementia?**

Part One

I begin this chapter with a kind of a riddle from the neurologist Oliver Sacks. I invite you to try to solve it and keep returning to it over the course of the book to see if it means any more to you:

> A Who has a What –
>
> Will the What overcome the Who?
>
> Will the Who emerge through the What?
>
> Or will the two combine in a way that embraces and transcends the Condition?

The reason for this chapter is that I believe dementia is different from other conditions, and an understanding of this is essential to the messages carried by the rest of the book. Many illnesses with a strong medical component do have interpersonal aspects, and you can never discount the effect of mind on body and vice versa, but dementia is different in the degree to which this is significant, and I will try to spell out some of the implications later. There are, of course, different types of dementia, medically speaking, including Alzheimer's, Vascular and Korsakoff's, but from the point of view of communication and relationship they have more in common than they are different.

For a long time what was called 'the medical model' held sway. Everything was put down to shrinkage of the brain, plaques and tangles, so that the condition was invariably spoken of in terms of problems – with reasoning, memory, carrying out practical tasks, orientation and various physical effects.

A definition I came across recently in an early textbook used all of the following words: 'degenerative', 'incapable', 'disintegration', 'adrift', 'disturbed', 'dislocation', 'regresses', 'ailing' and 'helpless'.

Tom Kitwood, the most significant psychologist in the dementia field, characterised this viewpoint as 'person with DEMENTIA' but strove to redress the balance with 'PERSON with dementia'. His discussion of the condition, by contrast, concentrated on identifying a number of needs to be met, amongst them 'comfort', 'attachment', 'identity', 'inclusion', and 'occupation'.

Here we find the negative and positive attitudes to dementia starkly opposed. Focusing on the former results in the terrifying image which many people have of the condition. Focusing on the latter provides the foundation for hope and practical advances.

But the phenomenon is even more complex than I have

yet allowed, because dementia affects no two people alike. Just as everyone without the condition is different, so those who develop its characteristics do not do so in the same ways or at the same pace. Each individual is the sum of their personal characteristics and experiences of life prior to its onset, and this affects how they progress. It makes prediction difficult and all talk of 'stages' – where professionals have classified aspects of the development of the condition into discrete phases and listed all the characteristics a person going through that phase is likely to display – is rendered meaningless. Many supporters speak of how the unexpected occurs in the lives of their loved ones, sometimes to astonishing effect, and I can demonstrate this from my own experience.

On visiting a care home, I was told by the manager, 'It's no use talking to Mabel today – she's away with the fairies'. I spoke with other residents until, some time later, Mabel approached me. 'May I ask you a question?'

'Of course,' I answered.

'Is there a moment between birth and death when one becomes more important than the other?'

There was a long silence. 'I'm sorry, Mabel, I can't answer your question, it's too profound.'

'That's alright. I just wanted you to know that that's what I was thinking,' she said. I returned to the home manager, told her the story, and added, 'If Mabel's away with the fairies, I want to join her.'

Of course, many people report problems which they find difficult to cope with, whether they are a person with dementia or are supporting someone. These include: getting lost in a familiar place; becoming over-assertive in company, or wanting to withdraw from socialising; spending long periods searching for or sorting items; sleeplessness; and incontinence. These must not be glossed over.

I have given an outline of the condition and indicated the challenges it poses us, both in terms of understanding it and in helping others to live with it. But it may still not be clear how great a challenge it poses for those in a supporting role. Because of the strong interpersonal component of the condition, we have a crucial task in helping people to adjust to their circumstances, but it also casts us in **the role of helping to create the atmosphere in which dementia flourishes.** The awareness that those around the person have a huge responsibility to avoid exacerbating the situation can come as a real shock, but this is a necessary shock we need to experience if real progress is to be made.

You may be asking: how is it possible for us to be, metaphorically speaking, carriers of this thing? Tom Kitwood frames his answer to this question in the form of a series of examples of what he calls 'malignant social psychology'. He doesn't mean by his use of this term to imply that any mistreatment is intentional, only that it occurs through lack of awareness of the effects of certain actions. He lists seventeen of these in total, including:

Treachery: deceiving the person to get them to do what you want

Disempowerment: not allowing a person to carry out a task they are capable of performing themselves

Infantilization: treating an adult as if they were a young child

Ignoring: speaking of a person in their presence as if they were not there

Outpacing: moving or speaking at a speed beyond the other person's capability

Mockery: making fun of another's incapacity

Objectification: treating a person as if they are a piece of dead matter, without feelings

Disparagement: telling another person they are worthless and damaging their self-esteem

We shall meet some of these ideas in the course of these pages.

It is almost impossible to read a book about dementia without coming across the phrase 'challenging behaviour'. What is meant by this is that people challenge us sometimes with the way they speak and act. We must understand that they are not choosing to do so; in almost every instance they are reacting to the inadequate (malignant) way in which we are behaving towards them. That is a hard nut for us to swallow.

Joanne Koenig Coste puts the case succinctly as follows:

> It isn't Alzheimer's that takes away a person's dignity, it's other people's reactions that do it.

On the positive side, Kitwood proposed the concept of 'personhood' – the idea that we should all concentrate on reinforcing, by our words and deeds, the person's sense of self. He also suggested that, if we could get things right, time and time again, we might even be able to imagine a situation where the condition recedes. This he called 'rementia' – perhaps an impossible goal to achieve but one towards which we should all be striving.

On a further positive note, if we can hang on to the idea that if we try our best to understand, to be patient, to develop our capacities for empathy and love, we really cannot be expected to do more. And, despite the difficulties, there are rewards too. John Zeisel in his book '*I'm Still Here*' devotes a chapter to what he calls 'The Gifts of Alzheimer's'. Amongst no fewer than 39 which he identifies are the following:

Emotional openness to others

Having a sense of humour

Enjoying the moment

Seeing others for who they are

Going with the flow

Greater insight

Knowing my work is 'good' work

We shall see some of these too in the course of subsequent chapters.

Part Two *Other Voices*

There is such a range of opinions and ideas to be covered here. I have decided to represent it by two accounts, one from Richard Taylor, whom we have already met in Chapter One, and the other from a supporter. Both speak eloquently from their respective viewpoints. Here is Richard's account of the experience of Alzheimer's disease:

> Right now I feel as if I am sitting in my grandmother's living room, looking at the world through her lace curtains.
>
> From time to time a gentle wind blows the curtains and changes the patterns through which I see the world. There are large knots in the curtains and I cannot see through them. There is a web of lace connecting the knots to each other, around which I can sometimes see. However, this entire filter keeps shifting unpredictably in the wind.
>
> Sometimes I am clear in my vision and my memory, sometimes I am disconnected but aware of memories, and other times I am completely unaware of what lies on the other side of the knots. As the wind blows, it is increasingly frustrating to understand all that is going on around me, because access to the pieces and remembering what they mean keeps flickering on and off, on and off.

Demonstrating a different perspective, these are the words of Caroline Brown, both of whose parents were diagnosed with dementia:

> It feels like I have been asleep for six years. The transition from daughter to mother to carer for my parents has taken its toll. That, frankly, is too heavy to bear at times. I have

worn the cloak of numbness, and no amount of prodding will dissolve it. That is until my awakening. The realisation of all that I had was missing, hit harder and shattered the numbness into a million tiny pieces.

I am wide awake and recognise the choice I have: to collapse under the grief that is Alzheimer's, that bit by bit grabs who my mum was but develops into the strength and dignity that even sitting in her wet incontinence pad could never take away.

I choose to love and to be loved and to know that her Alzheimer's will push me to make a difference to those who cannot know what it is like, to raise that awareness banner in the most subtle of ways because when I shout no-one hears.

Yet when I tell the story of who she is and what she has done to and for me, many will hear, many who will resonate with the helplessness of holding onto what once was but never will be again... and if we choose, the future can be better than anything that ever was in the past.

For ego and personality and power and control exist where human nature lives.

She gave all of that away to make room for what we now share.

Here in our new world where humility and spirituality and complete acceptance live, you cannot but be moved.

I choose awakening to what I can have now and not what I will never have again. The past – that is where it belongs.

I want to live and be fully awake in the now.

Thank you, awakening – I have arrived!

End Note

Without understanding that dementia is an interpersonal as well as a medical condition, we shall never realise that this gives us the priceless possession of being able to influence its development through the quality of our caring. If we succeed in this aim, we shall give good experiences to the person, and to ourselves as well.

Descartes, the famous philosopher, coined the phrase 'I think, therefore I am'. Stephen Post, the American ethicist wants that changed in relation to people with the condition to read:

'I feel and relate, therefore I am'.

CHAPTER THREE **Removing the Walls of Fear**

Part One

Fear is something we all have to overcome when we encounter someone with dementia for the first time. Or when we realize that someone close to us may be showing signs of the condition. It can take a number of forms:

- Fear of the unknown, where we come up against characteristics or situations we have never encountered before
- Fear that we may be hurt physically and/or emotionally by another person
- Fear of powerlessness: that we will be found wanting, that we will fail in the task with which we are confronted
- Fear that what is happening to the person before us may happen to ourselves in course of time

We may not be fully aware of the cause of our fear – it may be a mixture of these and other anxieties. It may not be possible for us to allay fully any of these fears. There are strategies we can adopt, though, which may help us with each of them to a greater or lesser degree. One thing is certain: if we cannot conquer them we shall be severely hampered in attempts to help or relate to the person in a meaningful way.

First, and most importantly, it is certainly true that familiarity can lessen the anxiety state. I don't mean that we can ever reach the situation of being able to take dementia for granted, but it can begin to seem less strange in the course of time.

It is natural to be afraid of anyone who acts differently from ourselves. If we do not understand why they act as they do, it becomes difficult to empathise with them. They challenge our view of the world that functions according to a set of rules, and change it into something incomprehensible and hostile. Here, surely, is the basis for the stigma that people have to endure, a situation made worse by the way we often talk about the condition and how the media exploit it. It is important to recognise that just as we are challenged, so are those who are going through the experience, and their struggle to make sense of it will be far more stressful than our own.

My introduction to people was sudden. I was shown into a unit of thirty people with dementia, told I would get nothing out of any of them, and the door was locked behind me. I knew nothing about the subject, and had never before met anyone with the condition. At first I was bewildered and felt alienated: why were these people acting in these ways, and how would I ever understand what they were saying? But as I lived alongside them my confidence grew. At the end of a week everyone was clear to me as a unique and lovable individual. The psychologist Tom Kitwood spoke of seeing the person not the disease, and I understood this before I ever heard him say it.

The fear of being hurt is lessened by the number of occasions on which it has not occurred. In my work I have had the privilege of meeting hundreds of people in many different situations (day centres, care homes, hospital wards, and in their own homes), and with different degrees of communication difficulty, and though I have found some of these encounters upsetting, the vast majority have proved life-enhancing.

It is true, however, that after about five years of one-to-one encounters, the emotional effect gradually crept up on me. One day I found I could not enter through the care home front door. I went to a counsellor. I thought I was having a 'breakdown'; she said I was having a 'breakthrough'. She also described it as 'a crash course in spiritual development'. The experience of encountering so many different people who were struggling with the changes they must come to terms with had changed me too: my emotions were nearer the surface, and this was something I must plan for in my subsequent work. I paced myself, and took time for reflection. I am sure this applies to everyone: respite is an important principle.

Fear of failure is, without doubt, the most likely to be realised of all these fears: there is no way that one individual can find the perfect answers to all the questions that will be raised by communication and relationship. The best you can hope for is that you will become more confident, and that the success rate, insofar as this is something that can be measured, will improve. A degree of humility is necessary, and the bar should not be set too high in the first place, so that when the special moments occur, as I am sure they will, you can take strength from them.

Finally, no-one can be sure dementia may not be something they will experience personally. Concentration on the positives will erase parts of the bleak picture which other people and the media will paint. Rather than push this fear under, it is better to bring it out into the open. One of the best things we can do for ourselves is to make plans for how we wish others to behave towards us if we were to develop the condition; in particular, what we would like supporters to know about our likes and dislikes in case we are not in a position to help them. 'Be Prepared!' is not just a motto for Boy Scouts!

Chapter Nineteen is an attempt to help along the process referred to in the last paragraph.

Part Two *Other Voices*

Deborah Everett has worked as a Chaplain in a hospital in Canada, and she offers this advice:

> The powerlessness that may occur when caring for a person with dementia has a lot to do with the caregiver's inability to value other means of communication than just words... When we see only meaninglessness, commitment is often lost. Surrender to the mystery of the future means admitting the possibility of suffering. Real care for those affected by dementia only takes place when the walls of fear have been removed.

This is the first part of a story by Laura Beck, who is a care partner in Ithaca, New York. It is set in an American care home. Her father was a military man, and had always been formal and unbending:

> One day I paid my father a visit. In the advanced stages of Alzheimer's Disease, he was long past simply forgetting my name. He no longer walked or spoke. Instead he had a language all his own, composed of various sounds and frequently uttered at the top of his lungs.
>
> Fresh from his bath this particular morning, I found him napping in his room. He awoke suddenly, wide-eyed, wide-haired, singing a loud, rowdy chant of nonsensical syllables. This vision of him overwhelmed me. My first reaction when I laid eyes on him was to reject what I saw.
>
> This wasn't the father I once knew... and I wanted him back.
>
> I stepped out of the room, overwhelmed. I wanted to turn

and go, but something stopped me. I asked myself what I was afraid of. The answer was clear – I was afraid of this happening to me. Once I named my fear, I felt maybe, just maybe, I could push through it...

The second part of this story follows in the 'Other Voices' section of Chapter Seventeen.

The passage which follows is Kate Grillet on the reactions she and her husband Christophe found:

Fear seems to be the only explanation for the withdrawal of love and friendship we experienced. One day I must ask family and friends to try and explain this. I used to get very upset (still do) when they talked about him having 'gone long ago', when he was definitely still here, that he wouldn't know that being in a care home was different from home, that he wouldn't know me or any of them, so it didn't matter who was with him. 'Don't you spend 3–4 hours a day with your partner/beloved?' I asked. Puzzled response.

In his famous book *The Prophet,* Kahlil Gibran offers this understanding of the process we must undergo in offering support:

Your pain is the breaking of the shell that encloses your understanding.

Even as the stone of the fruit must break, that its heart may stand in the sun, so must you know pain.

And could you keep your heart in wonder at the daily miracles of your life, your pain would not seem less wondrous than your joy.

End Note

Fear can take a number of forms, and we must strive to overcome them all if we are to truly relate to a person. And we need to help people overcome their own fears as well as deal with our own. We must develop the practice of listening carefully to what they have to say. Here are some lines on this subject from someone with the condition:

I'm frightened.

I'm frightened of being caught in a current.

And now I'm going to ask you a question:

Would you like to live like this?

CHAPTER FOUR **Being Aware**

Part One

A woman with dementia asked me one day, 'Would you please give me back my personality?' It was an impossible request, because one person cannot achieve anything of that magnitude for another. It put me in a unique dilemma too, because I had got to know her rather well, and she came across as a strong-willed feisty individual.

It was the same woman who, on another occasion, asked, 'What is this lump of matter if you can't make sense of it?' Her first question was a cry for help. Her second raised fundamental questions about the condition: how does a person cope when the changes they are experiencing make them doubt their own competence to deal with living?

And, of course, how can we help them to maintain an equilibrium? And further, how are we to deal with the anxieties – in recognising ourselves as vulnerable human beings – which are raised when we come into contact with this characteristic?

Many of the people I have worked with have confronted similar predicaments, though not always so explicitly. These are examples of insight. Once it was thought that people with dementia did not maintain awareness of this kind but it has now come to be accepted that many do.

It may well be that awareness fluctuates, but as verbal ability declines, people may not be able to let us in to their inner worlds to share their perceptions so perhaps it is more consistent than we imagine. Of course, it would be convenient for us as supporters to assume that a person does not have awareness as this lessens our obligation to make attempts to understand and respond to their psychological needs.

The implications for communication are clear: providing regular opportunities for people to converse, and to unburden themselves where necessary, is essential. Time and time again I have persevered in the waiting game, to be rewarded by remarks which emanate from a deep well of feeling or are indicative of profound thought:

> My mind, my whole sphere of life is full. I was very fond of my life. It seems that I'm leaving it more and more. Oh dear, it isn't fair when your heart wants to remember!

And here is what someone said as we were nearing the end of a long and intensely personal conversation:

I'm tired, but I don't want to fall asleep because I'm thriving!

I want to end this section with some consideration of the part played by awareness when a diagnosis is made. If we regard dementia as a spectrum, then this event looms large and can have unexpected consequences for the individual. I have spoken to many people about how they received this verdict. Some people struggled hard to get a diagnosis, and it came as a form of reassurance, in that it was a confirmation of what was expected. To some people it came as a shock which plunged them into depression. To others it was rejected and triggered a period of denial. Some people would rather not have known, because reactions to it can often adversely colour the rest of their lives.

Much seems to rest on how the diagnosis is delivered. At the one extreme it was given as a bare statement and to the supporter, not directly to the individual. They went home in a daze, got online, and read up all they could. The result was that both the person and their supporter were scared by the medical information they found. Clearly the doctor took no account of the part awareness might play in this process.

Others report that the diagnosis enabled them to find a fresh resolve and start planning the rest of their lives. This could be the result of the way in which the diagnosis was communicated, or that the person and their supporters already felt positive about how they would handle the outcome. Many of these people start filling the coming months and years with a variety of activities – the kinds of things one has always wanted to do but never got around to accomplishing. Another aspect was making arrangements for a time when one might not be so able to cope with some of life's demands, sensible strategies for one's latter days, in other words.

What seems common to all the accounts I have been given is the view that a diagnosis should be accompanied by a support system which helps people cope with the consequences. Of course family members and friends are part of that system, perhaps the most important part. The consistency and quality of what we offer will call upon our reserves of love and strength. We in turn can receive assurances from the growing number of insightful personal accounts of the opportunities which the condition presents. Some of these are to be found in these pages.

Part Two *Other Voices*

Here is an example of a humorous expression of awareness. It comes from Kim Zabbia's book about her mother:

> Mom leaned over to her granddaughter and said jokingly, 'Don't listen to your Mama. She's the crazy one, not me. What're you playin'?'
>
> 'I was trying to play Solitaire,' Kate said, 'but I can't. There's only fifty cards. I don't have a full deck.'

'That's okay, baby,' Mom grinned. 'I don't have either.'

And here is an extract which raises the possibility that there may be insights which are beyond expression in language. It comes from Michael Ignatieff's novel *Scar Tissue*; his mother has Alzheimer's and is dying:

> I had arrived at that moment, long foretold, hopelessly pre-pared for, when Mother took the step beyond herself and moved into the world of death with her eyes wide open.

There follow two reactions to receiving a diagnosis. The first is by James McKillop, a member of the Scottish Dementia Working Group, an organization made up of people with the condition, devoted to changing attitudes and improving services:

> Being told of the diagnosis at the right time, in the right place, by the right person who has thoughtfully allowed plenty of time for explanations and any questions is essential... Most people can start to confront a problem once they know and understand what it is. If not told the blunt truth, or if the issue is fudged, you are still in the dark, weaponless, fighting the unknown.

Rebecca Ley, in an article about her father describes an aspect of the dilemma raised by diagnosis:

> Sometimes it's better not to label the no-man's land between health and illness, especially when it involves an individual's loss of freedom. And confidentiality is important – there is only so far that concerned family members can go in expressing opinions.

However, I don't think anyone spent enough time properly appraising him or taking our worries seriously. There needs to be a hand there to catch those who are freefalling.

Kate Grillet speaks of her life with Christophe:

> Our experience of the diagnosis – memory problems, confusion, anger, 'unreasonable behaviour' (which was quite reasonable when you think about it), tests, brain-scans, the dismal predictions Christophe made about himself, having seen his Mum's decline, the neurosurgeon's unsympathetic manner. And we were cast adrift: no help or advice, no information about what to expect or how to respond, for about eight-ten years. I read books and eventually went to carers' groups. All this needs to change. The supporter needs supporting too, right from the beginning.

Helen Finch is a family carer with whom I have worked alongside her mother. In conversation with me, she reflects on the kind of support that is needed:

> JOHN: Can I ask you – because I know you have strong feelings about this – what does the person who is developing dementia need from other people? I don't mean services, I mean what do they need emotionally from others?
>
> HELEN: I think what they need is an acknowledgement of what has happened to them. And I think that people should be honest with them. For example, if a doctor has done a brain-scan and there are clear signs of deterioration, might it not be appropriate to actually in some way explain that?... I think too there needs to be some kind of a listening service, whether a counsellor or a doctor, and by their families,

perhaps in group sessions. It may well be that there's a place for groupwork with families in the early stages.

JOHN: That's for the people with the condition *and* their families? To get them all together, rather than taking their families on one side and counselling them?...

HELEN: As a group, as a family, yes, everyone. Because I think it is possible to get value out of counselling if they were to seek help. But maybe there is a place for both – for the person with dementia to be counselled individually, professionally. Also for group therapy for the whole family. And in this way everybody has a chance to talk through the problems. Our family was very lucky, we were able to talk things through together with mum to some extent, but even so I'm not sure it was enough.

End Note

Our attitude to awareness in the person is central to how we communicate with and relate to them. If it is not in the forefront of everyone's minds at the time of diagnosis, many upsets and misunderstandings can follow. It may reduce their chances of making use of whatever services are available, and lead to a failure on our part to address their emotional needs. In particular we need to cultivate an awareness in ourselves that when a person is silent this does not necessarily indicate a lack of insight on their part into who and where they are. As one lady said to me after a long period of wordlessness:

I'm thinking when I'm not saying anything.

CHAPTER FIVE **Maintaining Relationships**

Part One

Given the emphasis I have put on the supporter's role in Chapter One, the current one is obviously a key chapter. I believe the way we react to a person who begins to show signs of confusion can affect their wellbeing and even the pace of development of the condition. If we are contemptuous or dismissive of problems as they arise, this can create tension and instability in the relationship. If we are patient and adopt an empathetic approach, this can calm anxieties and create a supportive atmosphere.

I see I have used this word 'empathy' again without properly defining it. What I have in mind is the capacity to see things temporarily through another's eyes. This involves a lack of self-consciousness and a willingness to reach out emotionally to another in an attempt to understand their situation. It does not inhibit action in the way that 'sympathy' does, which suggests an emotionalism which is fundamentally unhelpful. Empathy is probably the single most important quality we can develop if we wish to maintain and even develop a relationship with someone with dementia.

Although there may be instances with the less common dementias of changes in the way a person presents caused by physical factors, as a rule it is better to assume that it is failings in our attitude that sparks off behaviour that is often labelled as 'challenging'.

It would surely be helpful to regard the onset not as the start of an inevitable decline but as an opportunity for fresh experiences and new ways of being. There are a number of accounts by supporters that bear witness to the lasting benefits of a positive approach established early on.

We need to be taking the pressure off the person with regard to reasoning and remembering, and to transfer our attention to ensuring their emotional stability. It is, of course, a challenge to both parties, but I am sure it will prove fruitful to reach a mindset in which we see this as a shared journey. It has the potential to be mutually rewarding as both grow into a new understanding and intimacy. The emphasis subtly changes from a spectrum which embraces before and after, to one that focuses on the moment. Chapter Sixteen explores this concept in more detail.

One aspect which can be difficult to deal with is that of sexuality. In normal ageing there may well be fluctuations in this area of personal relations, but dementia can cause some unforeseen changes: feelings may appear to diminish or to intensify, and there can be every gradation in between.

Danuta Lipinska is a counsellor who has worked a lot with people one to one and in groups. She has also reflected a great deal on the subject of sexuality in later life. She tells the story of a group she was running in which:

> One demure, frail-looking 86-year-old woman replied
> 'I'm a sixteen year old sex maniac inside this body, but no

one believes me!' The reaction of the group: embarrassed laughter, some whoops of delight, a couple of shocked stares and 'Good for you's'...

If you have previously been in a sexual relationship with the person, your own feelings may undergo a change. This is an aspect which tends to get neglected because it is difficult to talk about. If it proves impossible to discuss this with your partner, you may need to find another sympathetic person to confide in. Bottling these things up can only lead to greater distress.

It is unsurprising that out of need and a possible overflow of feelings (often maternal) some people respond positively to soft toys, especially dolls. Opinion is divided over whether this is something that should be encouraged. My own attitude is that if this is a manifestation of the playfulness I describe in Chapter Fifteen then this is fine; in which case the person will perfectly be able to discriminate between the real animal or baby and the toy. Where it becomes a substitute for real human interaction, then I think the practice becomes more problematic.

Mary was a care home resident I grew into a relationship with over a number of months. What follows is a reflection of the intimacy achieved by looking at a picture of the two of us interacting:

In the photograph we are standing in the unit, my left hand clasping yours. I, being much taller, am leaning forward, our heads are almost touching. We are laughing; your eyes are closed, with the intensity of the feeling, it seems. It is a shared joke, but since you have little language left, it may be something we have seen and identified. Or it may be that one of us has thought of something and the merriment has spilled over onto the other. As always, there is a complicity that goes beyond words.

Bodies play a big part in our relationship: we hold and hug and kiss. We are always on the move – dancing or walking – exploring our environment. You never seem to tire of new places and faces; or rather, the old places and faces seem to you ever-new.

Photographs are amongst your favourite things. Your face mirrors the feelings they evoke in you, and you keep up an appropriate commentary. I can tell that by the tone of your sounds. Your discourse is full of exclamations.

Your gestures are full of exclamations: when I come on the unit and you see me in the distance you approach, always pointing, pointing. And I do the same. Until our fingers meet and intertwine. You keep saying 'Oh you!' over and-over, as if you cannot believe your good fortune. I cannot believe mine.

Writing this I realise I hardly know anything about your past life. What we have is all in the here-and-now. It is enough.

Part Two **Other Voices**

Cary Smith Henderson is an American who has written a book about his dementia:

Well, if you're like me, I'm not sure you're thinking a

whole lot, but you have a lot of feelings. Everything we do is just full of feelings.

Frena Gray Davidson is also an American author:

In many ways the deepest revelation of the Alzheimer journey is that it is a kind of passage from the mind into the heart.

Kate Grillet describes her personal journey in these terms:

I became exhausted from lack of sleep and stress, and easily exasperated; but I continued to care for Christophe through what Oliver James calls 'the tipping point', and out the other side, and then I redeveloped a loving interest and a new level of tolerance (I gradually became accustomed to and unworried by Christophe's incontinence rather as I did when my children were little). I think I became calmer, but tireder and sadder, but there were so many rewarding moments too; it's a very bumpy road full of potholes and trip-wires.

Kate also comments on the sexual aspect:

When he was in the care home I longed to bring Christophe home, often, and wished they had had a double bed so that we could snuggle down together. I asked about staying with him and this was thought very strange with an incontinent man. I thought of him as my lover until the day he died, and still do.

Here is another part of the conversation with Helen Finch, quoted from in Chapter Four:

JOHN: This leads me to a very difficult question, which I

think is crucial. You have seen what dementia has done to your mother: robbed her of a whole range of capacities. Do you still see her as an adult, or has she become a child to you?

HELEN: Well I'm not sure I perceive anyone in such a black-and-white way. However, I still see her as my mother, and in that sense as an adult. What is difficult over a period of time is holding on to the person she was. But though some of her behaviour could be considered 'child-like' I don't see her as a child.

When you were younger your mother was a person you looked up to, that you turned to when you were in trouble. That is particularly true of my mother because she was always willing to listen... somebody you could use to sound out ideas. So it feels uncomfortable that her capacity for that is severely lessened. It is still possible for me to confide in her, that maternal bit is still there. But dementia makes it hard in so many ways. The first time I bathed her, for example, was absolutely shattering, I had to leave the bathroom and go downstairs and cry – it just didn't seem natural, that's the only way I can describe it.

JOHN: It confounds all expectations of role, doesn't it? But that's no different, is it, from any child becoming an adult and having to help an aged parent who has become physically incapacitated – it has nothing to do with dementia necessarily?

HELEN: No, it doesn't but...

JOHN: But it isn't just that, because she isn't just, or maybe at all, physically incapacitated?

HELEN: I am sure there is an extra dimension in this, because all sorts of other parts of the relationship which might be sustained throughout physical illness are more difficult to maintain because of the dementia.

JOHN: Talking about the feeling thing, because that is what ultimately binds people together, do you experience any difficulty in feeling close to your mother?

HELEN: No.

JOHN: Has it affected the closeness in any way?

HELEN: Yes it has. When any change takes place, and certainly any change that involves loss, there are a lot of negative feelings engendered, but I think there are positive aspects as well. In some ways dementia has brought us closer, certainly in a more open and physical manner. My mother, you see, was not highly demonstrative.

And there's another aspect: you are thrown back on a much more fundamental level of relating, in which you can't rely upon speech as you did, so you are concentrating with all your might on the kinds of communication we both relied upon when I was small.

End Note

Some relationships are long-lasting but dementia changes them; they may become more difficult, or they may deepen. We must be prepared for possible developments. New relationships can form, and quickly. A woman said to me:

If you'll still be here when I get back, that'll please me – I'll put a tick by your name.

A man said to me:

> There are not men here like yourself, men that you can talk
> to. If anyone asks you, say that you're my brother.

CHAPTER SIX **How Are You Managing?**

Part One

Some years ago I went to work in another country where
I lived alone in company accommodation. So it seemed
quite appropriate that a member of staff should come up
to me and ask 'How are you managing?' I immediately
understood their use of that last word to mean 'coping'
and answered them in the same terms.

Earlier that day I had been talking with another member
of staff and she had used the word in a quite different
sense. We were discussing approaches to communication
and she had described her work as 'a passion'. She talked
about how she always tried to respond to someone in as
spontaneous a way as possible, whilst at the same time
holding in her mind all that she had learned about that
person through previous encounters. So it came as something of a shock when she suddenly spoke of 'managing
challenging behaviours'. At that instant two philosophies
collided, and I was forced to reflect, not just on the term
'challenging behaviour' (already mentioned in Chapter 2),
but on the various meanings of the word 'manage' and
how our interpretations affect our practice.

I begin with the situation she and I were in at the time. It
is true that she had come to my office and we were facing

each other across a desk. But we had agreed the time and place of meeting, we were both eager to hear each other's stories, I was not formally her 'manager', and the desk was not a barrier between us but an object on which we could lean our elbows! We respected each other's space, and the space in each other's heads, and were free to converse or disengage at any time.

We went on to imagine an interaction with someone with dementia. Would the same equality operate? Or was there, consciously or unconsciously, the exercise of power on our part which amounted to dominance? We acknowledged how easy it is to adopt a posture which conveys the message of mastery. Or a tone of voice calculated to put the other person at their ease, whilst, perhaps, we fed them the idea of a course of action we wanted them to follow. Here we were aware of entering the area of Kitwood's 'malignant psychology'. Could this be an example of what he called 'Treachery'?

The conversation with my colleague ended, but my thoughts ran on. There were whole aspects of this power issue we had not even touched on, such as the personal motivation of the supporter, and the effects of the institution in which the interaction took place.

But staying on the level of power relations in the one-to-one situation, I realised I had completely overlooked the non-verbal. It is so easy and convenient to ignore this, because it is an area where those of us without dementia could actually be at a disadvantage.

Although experts say a major part of every conversation is non-verbal we tend to take it for granted. Confronted with someone whose verbal abilities have deteriorated, we have a choice: either we continue to concentrate on words, expecting little in return. Or we attempt to meet the person on their own terms, using the full vocabulary of sound, touch, body language, eye-contact etc to carry the messages (see Chapter 9 for a discussion of these).

This latter is a risky business, and can engender powerful feelings of inadequacy in us. Good. Don't we need these to redress, in however small a way, the balance of power so overwhelmingly weighted in our favour on most occasions?

If we can bring ourselves to embrace the non-verbal we shall be humbled by the experience. We have to learn to live with our lack of fluency in this unfamiliar world, and to take our cues from another who may, of necessity, have become far more accomplished in conveying and appreciating expressive subtleties. If a person is allowed to lead an interaction it may be an enjoyable and fulfilling experience for them.

This is one of the real and deep and challenging aspects of dementia. Consideration of it, and our past performance, can make us feel uncomfortable. I don't wish to hide the fact that, however enlightened our motives and earnest our intentions, we may find it difficult to achieve consistently such empowerment of the person.

Part Two *Other Voices*

Here is a woman with dementia speaking:

> I'm not going to ask for help. They've told me, I'm not to ask. They told me up the corridor. So I'll do as others do: I'll just go to sleep... They don't give you a chance: if you do this you'll get that; if you do something else you'll get the other.

And here is another woman complaining of what Kitwood calls 'Ignoring' (one of his categories of 'malignant social psychology'):

> Some people when my husband and I are together, they refer to me as 'her', not as 'us' or 'them' or 'you two'. It's like I'm there but they can't see me... And it's so aggravating – I want to stick my tongue out and say 'I have Alzheimer's but I can still comprehend and speak for myself most of the time'.

Helen Finch, speaking with me, makes a point about equality in relationship in the following words:

> HELEN: It feels important to treat a person as you have always done, and my feeling is very strong that that applies not just to my mother but to everybody that I meet who has dementia. We must try and communicate at a level that is no different from what it would be with anybody who *hasn't* got dementia – that feels to me like a fundamental principle.

> JOHN: Has it got something to do with dignity?

> HELEN: Absolutely. And one of the things that is most

distressing, I feel, is that occasionally there have been times when people have spoken to my mother in a way that was somehow different from the way they would have spoken to her if she hadn't got dementia. I find that terribly upsetting.

End Note

I need to remind you (as I constantly have to remind myself) that when a person is beginning to develop problems in making themselves understood, the task we face as supporters is even greater, particularly because it is more hidden. When someone cannot find a word, or has difficulty in completing a task, it is so easy (indeed almost second nature) for us to supply what is missing or take over the activity. In these instances we need to realise that we are robbing them of the opportunity to act, and rubbing in their inadequacy in a hurtful manner. That is why the question 'Who's in charge?' needs to be asked constantly, however painful coping with the answer may be. One person with dementia said to me:

> Everybody says 'You can do it.' Of course I can do it! But if I'm never given the chance...!

CHAPTER SEVEN **Hanging onto Memory**

Part One

Most people connect changes in remembering with dementia, so it may hardly be thought necessary to emphasise this aspect. It is important, however, to realise that it is also a characteristic of normal ageing. Where ordinary forgetfulness and dementia overlap is a grey area, and this is one of the reasons that diagnosis is by no means an exact science.

'My memory, it slims away,' one lady vividly described the process to me. But we have to distinguish between different kinds of memory – some don't 'slim away' as easily as others. Memories in the body of how to carry out certain tasks may be resilient till later on. Those associated with emotions can be very powerful, and recall is often assisted by a picture or a smell or a sound (music especially). Memories which can deteriorate include those for facts and figures (highly valued in our society), and those for putting names to faces. Memory is also very variable. Mental or physical wellbeing or confidence can play a part, and drawing a blank on one occasion may be succeeded by a surprising access of detail on another.

Reminiscence is the attempt to stimulate a person's recall by the use of photographs, objects, films, music etc. It is usually early memories that are being tapped into in this way. A strong reminiscence movement has built up in Europe, America and Australia to encourage people to share their memories, but this can prove a double-edged sword. One lady complained, 'The old days are baffling me to get them right.' The attempt to coax somebody into accessing this storehouse can be problematical – focusing on an area where people experience frustrating deficits.

For another, it can provide peak experiences – one lady said, 'I've been playing in the House of Ages!' I wonder if she was referring to a reminiscence session?

It is a commonly held misunderstanding that our memory-bank is like a library of videos, and all we have to do is select one for replaying. In fact our recall of events is an active process, always a construction, and therefore inevitably affected by gaps, misinterpretations and inventions, so that no autobiographical account you may read will be telling anything like 'the whole truth and nothing but the truth'.

For people with dementia, this state of affairs may be even more unreliable. What with forgetfulness, distortions of time, the strong emotional pull of certain events and persons and language problems, the memories will often turn out to be only vague approximations to the past as understood by others. The questions arise: does this matter? And how should we cope with a narrative that appears to be full of false statements? I am sure that, as in other circumstances, correcting the person is counter-productive. You may only upset them and make them feel inadequate. And it is disrespectful. Whilst not actively agreeing to what is said, surely we should maintain an encouraging stance? Everyone needs to talk, and to be listened to, however unlikely the narrative may seem.

As a person's language problems increase, the situation may be reached where speech is minimal. It may become difficult, if not impossible, to know what (or even whether) someone is recollecting. Behind the blankness you encounter, there is a real person with a memory, which they may be accessing but are unable to share with you except at certain moments. There are instances of the barrier suddenly being broken through, to overwhelmingly positive effect.

The wife of a clergyman on the unit where I was working once asked me if I could help her husband to recall events of his life. For over an hour she fed me questions to ask him. There was no response. Then she addressed him directly 'Do you remember, darling, when at the age of eighty you went paragliding for the first time?' Suddenly he stood up to his full height and declaimed, as if he was back in the pulpit:

> There were three of us in the boat and I was the first to do it. It was the flying, it was the feeling free. And when I flowed like that I was astonished. And then I flew again: ONE, TWO, THREE! When are we going again?

Then he collapsed back in his chair. His wife was in tears. Her husband had resumed his personal preaching style, and he had temporarily regained verbal fluency – all, it seemed, in the service of some powerful surge of an emotional memory.

I once talked with a lady who used the expression, 'Memories that bless and burn.' This reminds us that many of us have things in our lives we would rather forget. So when we are encouraging reminiscence we must be aware that we may be touching areas that are uncomfortable, even traumatic.

One of the most upsetting aspects of forgetting is where a person fails to recognise a familiar face, or mistakes one person for another, often someone significant to them in their earlier life. Frequently the error is accompanied by a surge of emotion: the person knows that you mean a lot to them, but mistakes the connection. Maybe you could try going along with this, and take comfort from the significance assigned to you.

Of course some people shake their heads over memory-loss and suggest that it is the end of meaningful life as we know and experience it. But it is possible to take a more pragmatic view. I heard of one doctor who, when faced with a patient bemoaning his problems, proposed, 'Don't say your memory is failing, think "I am becoming a better forgetter."'

Part Two *Other Voices*

As you might imagine, with this subject I have a host of quotes clamouring for attention. The first is from Will Eaves, a supporter writing in a newspaper. For some people, the condition brings relief from having to confront the no-go parts of their past. He speculates on whether this applies to his mother:

> I wonder whether the loss of certain strands of my mother's identity was altogether a terrible thing. Her myth of origin was a source of terrific pride: it underpinned a sense of her individuality within the family. It also caused her continuing distress – and when that distress, with its

mixture of guilt and longing, disappeared, it seemed to me that she was free to inhabit a magnified present, whose possibilities were bright, sad and joyful.

The conserved aspect of memory packed up, like a hard drive. The dynamic component – the lit screen – flickered on.

The senses are a great stimulus to remembering, and Claire Craig, an occupational therapist, whom we will meet more than once in these pages, offers us this potent example:

The emotional power of the sense of smell should not be underestimated. The sensory nerves in the nose are directly connected to the limbic system, the emotional brain. Only the other day, a lady with dementia sat and wept, talking of her lost children. To many her conversation probably seemed out of context, labelled 'confused', yet I too had caught the subtle odour of baby oil in the air, probably in someone's shampoo.

Many supporters, like HJ here, tell stories of how memory can sometimes be jogged in inexplicable ways and something magical can occur:

It had been a good two years since my mother could recognise me. One day as I was sitting at her side visiting, she looked right at me. Her face brightened, and she called to her nurse, who came over. With a broad smile of motherly pride on her face, she said 'I want you to meet my son.' Then, she faded and went away again.

Joan Woodward tells the following story:

> My mother was staying with me while she was in-between residential homes. One morning, when I took her breakfast in bed, she demanded, 'Where's Joan?'
>
> I explained that I was Joan to which her reply was, 'Yes, I know. But I mean my Joan. She's much younger than you are but she's got more sense!'
>
> This amused me so much that it took the edge off the realisation that, for the first time, she hadn't recognised me.

On the troubled, and troubling, matter of painful recall, the psychologist Stephen Davies has the following advice to offer:

> People with dementia are just as likely as anyone else to have had traumatising experiences in their past. The decline of their everyday memory skills may render their coping methods less effective. Everyone who 'had a bad war' may experience some resurgence of these difficult times and people with dementia may communicate these memories in an unusual way, through action rather than language. Being able to talk about the war may be crucial to understanding a particular person with dementia but it is a finely balanced process, not without risk. However, if carefully managed and monitored and with the intimate involvement of carers, it can allow the disarming of painful memories.

End Note

Memory seems all-important to those of us who treasure

it, but some people seem to cope with only partial recall, and the lives of some others seem to be unaffected or even enhanced by the loss of this faculty. Sometimes people who still retain their memories want to keep them private, as this lady did, reproving me for my prying:

> I lived on a farm. I still do. It is higher up than this. I'd take you there but I wouldn't want to take you there to start with. IT IS MINE! IT IS MINE!

CHAPTER EIGHT **Listening to the Language**

Part One

A true story, I'm afraid. Some years ago I was invited by the editor of a book to write a chapter on communication in younger people with dementia. After I had accepted it I realised I'd never met any younger people! I decided to embark on a crash course in getting to know some people who fell into that category, and I enlisted the help of Alzheimer Scotland. That is how I came to find myself one afternoon in a tiny bedsit in the Leith district of Edinburgh. There was a bed on one side of me, and Alison, an Alzheimer Scotland worker, on the other. At the foot of the bed sat Bill, the man I had come to see.

I got out a list of questions and started to ask them. Each one was met with total silence on Bill's part. As I worked my way down the list I began to think that his communication problems were severe. Then suddenly he turned to Alison, and with a gleam in his eye, he asked, 'Shall we shut John up?' She clearly didn't know what to say. But Bill knew what he was going to do: on the bed lay his dressing-gown, and he picked it up and threw it over my head. For the next ten minutes (though it seemed like longer to me) Bill and Alison carried on a perfectly normal conversation, whilst I, sweating and confused, sat silent under the covering.

Then Alison ventured, 'Shall we let John out?' Bill lifted the corner of the garment and said 'You can come out now, you bugger, so long as you promise not to ask me any more of those stupid questions.' I promised, and was released. I could see him smiling: he had certainly enjoyed the joke at my expense. I wonder if Bill really appreciated how much he had taught me about the true nature of communication in those few minutes under the dressing-gown? There is a further moral to this story, though. When I got back to my office and looked through my questions I realised that by listening to his conversation with Alison I had received answers to everything I wanted to know.

Early signs of confusion can often show themselves in problems with language. At times vocabulary seems to have gone on strike, and either the words won't come or they emerge in an unconventional fashion. One lady I was conversing with put it this way:

> You and I, John, we speak the same language. Only you speak it straight and I speak it upside down.

This can be very frustrating for the person, and irritating

for anyone hopeful of understanding and providing an appropriate response.

It is impossible for me to provide you with a blueprint for interpretation, not just for **every** situation but for **any** situation. I can only give examples and some general guidance.

Here are some illustrations of speech in action. 'Who's in charge of the spare words?' a man asked me. The idea that someone's job could be to help one with language is a novel one, but it may indicate the importance of communication to someone experiencing difficulties, perhaps for the first time.

A lady said, 'You are words. Sometimes people give you words back, and they are all broken, patched up.' I think she meant that we are judged by the language we use. So her perception is that people are developing a low opinion of her because of her difficulty. She knows she isn't stupid, but feels that circumstances are making her seem so. And she is distressed by the lack of understanding shown by others.

Another characteristic which develops in some people, and which can puzzle the listener, is the use of symbolic language. I mean by this, words or ideas used to stand for others. For example, a man said to me 'Have you any openings? Have you got a guide? Could you come and turn a key in a lock for me? You'll not find my room. I've got... nothing.' It was pretty clear to me that he was not talking about somewhere he lived but about how he felt he was coping mentally. Many people, it seems to me, show insight of this kind.

Cathie Borrie, an American writer, has transcribed the sayings of her mother in a little book. When she asked her mother, 'What do you think about the sky?' the reply was:

> Oh I don't know about the sky, I don't really know about it. It's pretty beautiful but you have to wear gloves because it puts fingerprints on it and you don't want that.

Poetry is the language of feeling and frequently employs metaphor. There are a number of examples of this kind of language use found throughout this book. I believe they come from the emphasis on emotion rather than reasoning, which I have already referred to.

It may be that the creative aspects of language that we encounter come from a greater access to the unconscious mind. It's as if the brakes are off and the mind freewheels in ways which intellectual control restrains. One lady seemed to be referring to this when she said, 'I'm blethering, but it's all from beneath the surface.'

I promised you some general hints about the positives and negatives of verbal communication. Please regard these as suggestions, not a prescription!

- It helps to sit in front of the person rather than alongside them (and certainly not behind them). This enables you to maintain eye-contact. Obviously you need to be on the same level as well.

- Make sure the person can also see and hear you properly – with glasses on if they are worn, and with hearing aid working properly.

- Take time to listen. Make it clear that you have chosen to be there with the person, and that this time is for them.

- Make sure your facial expression and tone of voice are encouraging. You could try holding the other person's hand as physical reassurance, if this seems appropriate.

- If there are silences avoid filling them with chat – it could cut across the other person's attempts to gather their thoughts and words. The lady who said, 'You are words,' also said to me, 'You have the stillness of silence, that listens and lasts.'

- Where the other person is experiencing difficulty avoid stepping in to finish sentences. Let them – however haltingly – speak for themselves.

- Don't automatically encourage reminiscence – the other person may not want to talk about the past.

- In your own contributions use short, simple sentences.

- Try to avoid questions if they are likely to highlight memory problems. (Or if they can appear insulting!)

- Try using prompts to provide a topic of mutual interest – it could be a photograph or an object or a piece of music or a piece of film – but don't insist on a response.

People with memory problems sometimes ask the same question over and over, which can prove very wearing for the listener. Whilst you should not ignore the person after you have already supplied an answer, perhaps the most helpful strategy could be to develop the reply into other aspects suggested by the question so that a full conversation can ensue. Sometimes it may be necessary to direct the question into a different subject area by offering a stimulus which breaks the chain of repetition.

I don't regard providing a distraction as unethical, but conscious lying is definitely to be avoided. It is destructive of a relationship of trust, and in practical terms anyway can lead to situations where the person receives different answers from different people and becomes even more confused. The individual may also experience different degrees of awareness at different times, and this too can lead to confusion. Best is to confront the question head on, and try to work out what is behind it. It may then be possible to address the feelings which occasioned it.

Another characteristic often come across is where the person refers to him or herself in the third person. Kate Grillet used to tell Christophe's life story beginning 'Once upon a time...' He would comment, 'That sounds like Christophe.' And speaking of his own fondness for washing he would comment 'He likes a warm bath.'

Part Two *Other Voices*

Larry Rose is someone with dementia, and he is clear about what he wants of those communicating with him:

Praise, encouragement and a show of affection can go a long way in calming an Alzheimer patient. I can tell you from experience. It can be very upsetting, even frightening when I am speaking to someone that does not speak clearly or does not use direct sentences, uses slang, is unwilling to repeat and does not use a tone of voice that is warm and empathetic.

Helen Finch and I were discussing how much a person can comprehend:

JOHN: You know your mother so well, do you think she understands things you say to her?

HELEN: I'm not always able to tell, so this is a problem. I hope that I err on the side of assuming that she understands more.

JOHN: There seem to be two ways of looking at this. There are some who assume that because dementia robs people of intellectual capacity they will not be able to understand. And there are those who practise the big 'as if' – they say we must proceed 'as if' people are understanding more than they can show.

HELEN: I take the second view. It's so difficult, because you realise you may be wasting your time, or even creating further difficulties for yourself and stress for her. There is no way of knowing for certain. My own view is that if you get it right only some of the time in a conversation then it's worth it. One of the things that having a close relative with dementia has taught me is that you have to be brave enough to take risks.

Michael Verde is the President of an organization in Chicago called 'Memory Bridge', and he offers the following advice:

> The next time you communicate with someone who is not at his or her cognitive best, remind yourself of this: 'This interaction is not about me. This interaction is about someone who is seeking connection on terms that may not advance the interests or needs of my ego. I am going to go where your needs are taking you. I am going to be with you in that place, wherever and however it is. I am going to let my ego disappear now. I am going to love you in your image instead of trying to re-create you in mine.'

End Note

'In the beginning was the word,' says the Bible, and we certainly put a lot of stress on being fluent in our native language. Where a person is still able to find words to embody their thoughts and feelings we should make every effort to communicate with them verbally, and celebrate their often creative attempts.

In what spirit should we approach this activity? Follow Sue Sweeney and, 'Listen with the ears of your heart.'

CHAPTER NINE **Learning the Language without Words**

Part One

You know the expression 'at a loss for words'. Well, when faced with communication with someone with dementia, many of us are at a loss *without* words. Perhaps visiting a person in a care home or a hospital bed we find them staring into space. We don't know what to do, how to engage with that person. We find ourselves mouthing platitudes which occasion no response. We begin to wonder why we came and what to do. The answer could be to practice all that life has taught us about being non-verbal.

If you are a supporter of someone, from within or outside a family, then you may have seen a gradual loss of fluency of speech over a period. This will have given you more time and opportunity to practice your skills in this area, both in interpretation and in your own expressive potential.

Tom Kitwood, the psychologist, urged us all to become more proficient in 'the language without words'. He also suggested that those with dementia may be better at this than we are. Perhaps, of necessity, they have learned to 'read' our behaviour, and answer us eloquently in the same kind. If so, that is a matter for congratulation: we have found one of the areas in which people with dementia have the advantage over the rest of us.

I must admit that I have sometimes felt uncomfortable that I appear to be being 'seen through' by someone with dementia. Maybe all those little subterfuges I practice are counting for nothing, and my real motives are being exposed. This can work in reverse: the person with whom we are interacting seems transparent, and the essential person shines through. One woman with the condition

said to me 'I bet you've never been so near Nature before.'
I took this to mean: 'with me you get the real deal.' We
may or may not be comfortable with what is exposed,
but we must recognise that in instances where the verbal
may have been compromised, the non-verbal is doing the
truth-telling.

It may be helpful at this juncture to list what a non-verbal
vocabulary can consist of. I expect you will be surprised at
its extent and variety:

- Use of the eyes, including eye-contact and gaze
- Facial Expression
- Voice, including tone, pitch, volume, rate and rhythm of
  speech
- Touch and physical contact
- Body movement and gesture
- Placement of the body in relation to another person
- Dress, appearance and smell
- Timing and pacing
- Creative expression, including music, painting, dance
- Plus combinations of all of these!

One aspect of non-verbal communication which can
assume crucial importance is mirroring. This is where you
imitate what a person says, or the sounds they make, or
the actions they perform, in a spirit of confirmation and
support. It is a way of saying 'I am watching and listening,
I am with you, and I am trying to understand'. Of course
you may not fully understand, but you do in the sense that
your concentration is upon the person and their attempt

to communicate and you are acknowledging that fact. It is a form of encouragement for them and will usually lead to a further attempt on their part to get a message across. If you fail to respond in this way then the communication could fail at the first attempt.

Have you considered walking as a form of communication? It is surely not just a matter of travelling from here to there. There is much to be learned from where we choose to walk, and the particular expressive ways in which we accomplish this process. Unfortunately many people with dementia find this activity labelled as 'wandering'. In wards of hospitals and corridors of care homes one can often find people on the move, singly or in pairs or groups. Maybe this is the result of a lack of meaningful activity. Or they are looking for an exit. Another possibility is that it is a response to inner frustration – the inability to resolve tensions or confusions. We all know that when we are faced with an apparently unsolvable problem, taking exercise can serve to clear the mind and perhaps light upon a solution. A way to respond to someone's apparently tireless onward movement is to accompany them, and not just physically: companionship and compassion are precious gifts we can offer.

I could easily devote the rest of this book to examples of the non-verbal; instead I will draw your attention in particular to Chapters Thirteen and Eighteen, and offer two short, necessarily inadequate, descriptions of interactions which took place in the busy lounges of care homes:

Bronwen comes into the room looking for me and leads me to a chair. I ask her permission to sit. 'Yes' she says.

'Is there anything you want to say to me?' I ask. She puts a finger to her lips enjoining silence. I repeat the gesture to show that I have understood. She runs her right hand over the chair arm, and then massages my hand, and touches my face. We maintain close eye contact.

She takes my right hand in what begins as a greeting and turns into a game of shaking hands vigorously. She points to a vase of flowers and later to a scene outside the window. She nods and says 'Yes' and so do I. I am attempting to mirror everything she does, but I am hardly conscious of doing so.

Eventually, after eight minutes of intense silent inter-personal communication, in which we are both largely oblivious of anything or anyone in the room, she places my hands on the table. She appears exhausted, and closes her eyes; then opens them again and nods. 'Yes' she says. Then drops her gaze again. 'Wonderful' she murmurs.

It is only afterwards that I reflect that Bronwen has been in charge of the interaction at all times.

*

I enter the room and am astonished to see Jane propped up much higher in her bedchair than before, with her eyes wide open, taking in all that is going on. I almost do a double-take: is this the woman I had seen on two previous occasions?

I go over to her; she does not seem fazed by my approach. I draw up a stool, sit down and greet her. She smiles back.

At first both her hands are under the blanket. I remember how previously she had gripped my hand tightly, and want to find out if this is still the case. After about ten minutes I reach for a hand and begin stroking it.

All the time she continues observing her surroundings in a pleasantly relaxed manner. Her tongue is not exploring her gums as before, but she is silent. At one point she summarily withdraws her hand, and grins, as if to say, 'That caught you out'.

Then an even more remarkable thing happens. I realise that she wants to look at me, but not while I am maintaining eye-contact. So I look away for about ten seconds. I can see through the corner of my eye that she is scrutinising me closely. I slowly return my gaze to her face, giving her time to look away again.

This manoeuvre happens three times before I decide to play a trick on her. I look back abruptly and our eyes meet. She gives out a roar of laughter, and so do I, almost simultaneously, in the complicity of the joke.

Part Two *Other Voices*

The first two quotations here are about touch, and come from Raymond Tallis, a geriatrician, and Margaret Silcock, a social worker:

> Through touch, hand may speak directly, and exclusively, to hand. What speech, what new meanings may emerge in silence, when hand meets hand, when this master manipulator, explorer supreme, this peerless communicator, meets another like himself!

*

I remember once on a routine hospital visit walking through a ward when an old lady stretched out her hands, took mine and started turning them, over and over as if she was washing them. This went on until I must have begun to loosen my fingers and withdraw them for then she pulled them closer to hers and went on with her ringing movement. Finally she let my hands fall, gently murmuring 'Thank you... that's enough.' Whatever it was I had given her, I knew I couldn't have given it to her any other way.

In the next extract Claire Craig, an occupational therapist, describes how through gaze a man is able to enter fully into an interaction:

Jack did not speak but didn't need to – his eyes expressed far more than words could ever say. Humour, fun, mischief, pathos, pain, frustration. He would command our sessions together, directing my actions. I would walk into the room and his eyes would immediately look to the window, the bottom of the bed, the radio, willing me to act and I would respond, 'Would you like the window opening?' – a nod of the head, a smile. 'More bed covers, Jack? – no response 'Oh, should I move the covers back?'... Our silent conversations went on.

Heather Hill is a dance therapist in Australia. She has some wise words to offer on the subject of keeping on the move:

Walking seems to be a way to get back in touch with yourself. The feet are highly sensitive with multiple nerve endings and perhaps this serves to stimulate and reinforce our being. Possibly, too, the regular rhythm of our feet making contact with the floor gives us a reassuring rhythmic structure and a feeling of being held, contained by the ongoing regular flow of movement. Walking can help us think, but walking can also provide us with stimulation and a reminder that we exist.

The final quote comes from Caroline Brown, a supporter whom you have already met in the Other Voices section of Chapter Two. Her mother is in a care home:

I have just got back from helping my darling mum with her breakfast. Her eyes never left me and it looked like someone had switched a light on behind them. She was so beautiful – how can anyone experience so much where no words are used? How lucky I am!

End Note

Non-verbal communication assumes more and more importance where verbal language has declined. Many people seem to develop expressive and interpretative skills in this area, and we need to concentrate on improving our capacities if we are to continue with and develop our relationships with them. There are rewards awaiting us if we persevere: the theologian Ronald Rolheiser speaks of: 'the language of silent embrace'.

CHAPTER TEN **Telling Tales**

Part One

I'm hoping that the title of this chapter carries a double meaning: that of the stories we tell, and of the significance that we attach to them. We all have a need to speak about our experiences; it confirms our importance to ourselves, and we hope to convince others of the meaningfulness of our lives.

It is often said that in later life our need to make sense of what has happened to us grows more acute: a kind of summing-up is felt as an imperative. This is just as important for people with dementia, but they may need help to achieve this.

Some people manage to share their stories. Some, lacking significant others to fulfil the role of listeners, tell them to themselves, perhaps out loud. Some, having tried and failed to be heard, may have abandoned the attempt altogether.

The act of listening is not a passive one. Although you may avoid interrupting or contradicting and prompting as much as possible, you do have to listen intently, with both respect and curiosity. You should make it clear that you regard this as their time, and not allow yourself to be distracted by other tasks. If at the end of a session you feel physically and emotionally exhausted, then this is an indication that you have given as much as you can ask of yourself.

Amongst the powers of attention you will need are:

- Watching the eyes and face for expressive indicators and the body language.
- Listening to the tone and inflection of the language used; this can sometimes tell you as much as the actual words employed; indeed if the sentences come out confused these may be your only guides to interpretation.
- Responding quickly to changes of attention and mood; you may not be able to keep one step ahead of the person, but you will certainly lose them if you once allow yourself to fall behind (this is literally true if they walk about whilst continuing the narrative – you may need to walk with them in order to maintain the interaction).
- Providing physical reassurance where necessary. This will very frequently involve holding hands; not only does this provide demonstrable proof of your concern, but much can be told by the intensity of pressure exerted in return.

The amount of planning that should go into these sessions will be minimal. Through practice you can develop a confidence and spontaneity that can become instinctive.

Sometimes you may need to provide a stimulus to get a person started. A photograph or an object or a piece of music can be useful here. They need not be reminiscence items.

You may want to have a record of stories you are told. This would involve you in writing down, or recording and then transcribing, or videoing the person speaking. I have not found that these practices in any way inhibit the person. Rather, they confirm them in their own importance and assure them of your sincerity in carrying out the task.

Sometimes we encounter a kind of 'stream of consciousness' from the person. This is where the speech is continuous, and seems to move from one subject to another without any apparent connection between them. Or there may be an uncensored series of metaphors offered to us. Beth Shirley Brough, an Australian supporting her friend Reg, describes such occasions:

> To my shame, I was often far too slow to tune into what was the real and most important issue of the day. Once I learned to treat what he said as the relating of a dream, once I listened for images and took them very seriously, we were able to explore very deep reserves within each other.

Difficult though such monologues may be to interpret at times, they must still be valued.

All storytellers need an audience, but if they don't have one nothing will stop some people from telling stories to themselves. I have met a number of people who carry on a continuous conversation in the absence of a listener. This should remind us that telling a story is fundamentally a social act, and, even though you may not interrupt, or even contribute, and the narrative may be confused or repetitive, your presence there is crucial: nodding and affirming is an essential part of the process.

I have been privileged over the years to be the custodian of many stories and will offer two examples from much longer narratives. Lily spoke all in a rush, and when I wrote her story down (I had taken the precaution of recording her) I kept it all in one long paragraph to emphasize its headlong nature:

I'll give you a title for this – 'The Gift of the Gab'! It's all about people that have good talking experience and ability. I wouldn't say that I had it – that would be conceit. Don't bring the worst out in me or it'll be bad for both of us. 'The Gasp of the Gib' – that would be a better title! I had one sister Elaine, younger than myself. We went to St Henry's, then St Brigid's at lessons. I was better at playing at the bat and ball. My interior physical world was good. I never thought I'd be able to sit down and babble like this about my educational times. My father didn't see the point of me being pushed into study, dear boy. You're not rushing me, I know that I want to do this. I followed into the catering trade because that was the locality's business. Cadena in the first place. My mother was in catering, it was open to most people of ability. My colleagues'll be having a good laugh at me gibbering on like this, they'll say we've got a right one here!

You will have noticed that Lily is very conscious of what she is doing: almost every addition of a detail is accompanied by a comment on present circumstances. One has no reason to doubt the veracity of her account. However, with Oliver there is clearly a strong fantasy element in his story. Both Lily and Oliver employ humour, and Oliver is also aware that I may well end up laughing at his inventiveness:

> I'm a bit of a comedian, and I'll tell you why. I go to a
> certain place just up the town. And there's a man lying on
> the floor dead naked. And there's another bloke standing
> over him. And I see they're both well-built types. I go away
> and come back five minutes later and the naked bloke's
> been stabbed three times through the bloody heart! So I tell
> the police and they catch him. They're pleased with me, I
> can tell you. If you told anyone that story they wouldn't
> believe you!

Which of these stories is the more valuable? My answer
to that question is that I believe they are both of equal
importance to the teller. Lily is explicit about the significance of the process to her. Oliver indicates as much by
giving himself the central role in his little drama. Both are
engaged in the essential task, which must be repeated over
and over, of asserting their sense of self.

Part Two *Other Voices*

Here are the views of the playwright and novelist Michael
Frayn; I believe what he says applies to everyone:

> This is how we make sense of the world – through the
> stories we tell about it, to ourselves and others. People
> were surely telling stories long before they attempted
> strictly historical narratives that venture some kind of
> precise and literal mapping of what happened, and they
> are likely to go on doing so, in one form or another, for

as long as life endures. ... This is what a story can suggest – how people act, not like cogs moved by the machinery of circumstance, but as autonomous beings, on the basis of what they perceive and understand, and of what they invent for themselves.

This is the experience of a supporter and writer, Jane Crisp:

My mother's stories about herself have a proper narrative structure yet because she has Alzheimer's they are largely untrue, being mostly woven out of fragments drawn indiscriminately from real, fictional and fantasy stories. However, this becomes less of a problem if we consider stories like hers precisely as stories, which in all essential respects they are, and judge them much as we would a story in a novel or a film, or one told us by a friend. The relevant criteria would no longer be the literal truth or falsity of the details but such aspects as the credibility of the story line, the pleasure and amusement it gives the teller and their listeners, and the overall point of the story – the underlying message or thematic and metaphoric meanings it suggests to us. Similarly, by thinking of people like my mother as story-tellers, we can start to see them as performing a socially valid role rather than as simply being confused or mistaken about the facts; and we can also start to make better sense both of what they are doing and of the stories that they tell us. If we stick with closeness to reality as our primary criterion, however, we handicap the storyteller from the start and deprive ourselves of anything but a negative response to them.

End Note

Stories are the stuff of life and of relationships, and that applies as much to people with dementia as everyone else. We need to become good encouragers and listeners, and not to interrupt or criticize. Lily, whom we met earlier in the chapter, said, 'I must make up my story for myself.'

Jane Crisp gives us a one-sentence summary of the process:

Strategy number one is a general strategy, on which all the others depend – to value the fact that the person we care for is still interacting with us.

CHAPTER ELEVEN **Seeking the Spiritual**

Part One

When I had the stroke
The feeling crept up my body
like lightlessness
like I was a cloud high up
like I was going to float away
and I was getting lighter and lighter all the time

Since then
I haven't had a fear of dying
because I know that's what
it will be like

Don't be afraid of it
because the feeling was wonderful

That's the time
When my second life began
The reason God gave me a second chance
was so that I could make other people happy

*

Twice and twice over what I think is important. My hiding place now is one that I can stretch out to and run away to for a while.

Both these quotations from people with dementia seem to me to express spiritual states. Sylvia Roberts, the speaker of the poem I made from her words, has a clear faith which her physical predicament has only served to intensify. The second, anonymous person might be referring to her memories, but I got the distinct impression from speaking with her that she was referring to a private meditative world. On another occasion she specifically denied me access to it.

The spiritual is one of the most intimate aspects of the person, and seems to have these two main characteristics: that of adherence to a specific faith-system, and that of an individual philosophical approach. We need to accord equal respect to both life-choices.

For some people a certain set of tenets has guided their thoughts all their lives. In Western societies these have been predominantly Christian. For such individuals each new life-experience has tended to be referred to the principles and attitudes to life which stem from that particular orthodoxy. A faith can add meaning, perspective and a context to a life. But dementia can pose a challenge to even the most strongly-held belief system.

One of the earliest first-person accounts to be published was by American clergyman Robert Davis. He was a man of steadfast convictions, filled with a passion to promote the faith. At first panic and despair set in. Then he experienced a revelation: Christ spoke to him and urged him to cease struggling.

Another reaction sometimes encountered is that of rejection. An individual can take the onset of dementia personally, and angrily accuse God of having deserted them. This is a position which it is difficult for others to counter except by patiently emphasizing positive approaches. This is not made any easier if the supporter does not share the beliefs which the person is questioning.

Susan Miller, the American novelist, takes the view that her father's strongly held beliefs served him well. She wrote:

> He thought of this illness without ego, precisely **without** the sense of self and grief for the loss of self that would afflict me if I found I had Alzheimer's Disease.

Many people, while not subscribing to a particular creed, see themselves as having spiritual needs which must be met. The great milestones of birth, love, loss and death give rise to feelings in everyone which, whether they choose to recognise it or not, are occasions with strong spiritual implications. Dementia, experienced by the individual, and by their supporters, must surely now be added to the list of significant shared events in the lives of a large number of people.

Christine Bryden is speaking to those without the condition, but on behalf of those with it, when she asks for the whole issue to be widened out:

> Spirituality is not simply what religion we might practise; it is important for you to help us re-connect with what has given us meaning as we journey deeper into the centre of our being, into our spirit.

In my view the big question is this: does dementia have the capacity to engender change in the spiritual realm as well as in the physical and mental? Perhaps it does. It may even be the case that the very decline of reasoning ability releases in some individuals a new capacity for spiritual development. It certainly forces us to value the person in their essential self rather than for any other values (economic, political, intellectual) which society upholds as paramount; these values have a tendency to obscure qualities such as honesty, truthfulness and transparency. Dare we even admit to ourselves the possibility that people with the condition could show us the way to identify and cherish the fundamental values we all share? There are just too many accounts of special experiences by people with dementia and their supporters for us to ignore this phenomenon.

I have already indicated in this book my belief that in confronting dementia we are confronting one of the great mysteries of life.

It has been the traditional role of the spiritual in all societies and in all periods to confront mysteries of this kind. Science in our day, in attempting to meet the physical challenges of the condition, is also entering the unknown. We must not neglect what the spiritual approach has to offer us, though. And we should be listening to what people themselves can bring to our understanding in this sphere.

Part Two *Other Voices*

Here are the views of two supporters, Beverly Murphy and Deborah Shouse:

> If you believe in the concept of a soul, then you have to believe that the soul doesn't get Alzheimer's any more than it gets cancer. Maybe the soul has an awareness of life around it that transcends the body or the ability to communicate… Maybe, just maybe, our people have the unique experience of being able to live in two worlds, ours and a freer one that allows them access to insights and awareness we can't even begin to fathom.
>
> *
>
> I sink into my mother's face like she is a meditation. We smile at each other for a half-hour, something we have never done before, something that would be too intense, too personal in our earlier, rational life together. Then her eyes gently flutter shut. I feel like I've been on a mystical retreat. I feel a rich sense of renewal and hope.

And a further reflection from Caroline Brown, who contributed so memorably to Chapters Two and Nine:

> Seven years of challenges and gifts that are dementia. Mum has advanced Alzheimer's. Dad's vascular dementia and bowel cancer took him in November 2012. You might imagine the existential 'WHY?' – unanswered questions that resided in my heart and head, exhausting me in the process. This dementia thing almost swallowed me up whole, yet ironically it was the faith gift from these two wonderful parents that evolved my spirit in spite of diagnosis.
>
> My appetite for end-of-life care hosted my most spiritual conversation with dad, sensing and giving me courage to tell him it was ok to go to his God. We held hands and prayed the Hail Mary over and over. In a whisper, he told me he thought he was ready. Dad died the following morning. Something freed me to discover a most sacred relationship with mum. Spirituality is to be found in the most surprising of places. Especially within dementia... I invite you to explore it.

And more of the words of Christine Bryden:

> This unique essence of me is at my core, and this is what will remain with me to the end. I will be perhaps even more truly 'me' than I have ever been.

End Note

We need to be aware of the changes that may occur in the person, both in terms of traditional belief and in wider spiritual awareness. Sometimes this manifests itself in premonitions of another world; sometimes in the here-and-now of intensified relationship. One day a lady said to me:

> Oh I went look up in the sky and saw it shining there and said 'That is Life'.

> Are you going to take me to see the sun?

CHAPTER TWELVE Coming to our Senses

Part One

One lady I spoke with had a very highly developed visual sense. This is how she responded to the place where we were sitting:

> The scenery of this room, does it ever get changed? Some of the compositions are so good it would be tragic to part with them. Someone should photograph them before they get changed, or they could be lost for ever. But at the same time you need variety, don't you, or you've nothing to compare? This room should be filmed before it is too late.

Do you have a favourite sense? Do you prefer looking at things (flowers, paintings, landscapes)? Or listening (other people's conversations, night sounds, music?) How would you feel if one of these was seriously impaired? We only need recall what it was like to lose our senses of smell and taste when we had a heavy cold to know how unpleasant it is to be deprived in this way, and these are not the most important senses for keeping in touch with our world and those around us.

Many people, particularly older people, whether they have dementia or not, experience serious loss in one or more of their senses. I hardly need point out that this can cause significant communication problems between people and their supporters, as well as health professionals. It can tend towards people becoming marginalised and their opinions not being sought.

If we want to pay more than lip-service to the principle of inclusiveness we need to develop strategies which are both practical and compassionate. It is obvious that shouting at someone who is deaf is not only counter-productive but damages relationships. We need to be aware that a person who is already trying to cope with other changes in their ability to make sense of things may be doing this in the context of a sensory disability. Often their confidence will suffer a severe blow. Somehow we have to find a way of operating on a day-to-day basis which is reassuring to the person and tolerable for ourselves – not an easy equation to square.

For those without a visual problem, but with verbal comprehension and perhaps other sensual impediments, a Talking Mat might prove helpful. This consists of a textured object which is placed between you and the person. There are three picture faces at the top of the mat – happy, sad and puzzled. There is a selection of pictures representing different subjects or activities, and you ask the person to put a specific picture below the face that says what they feel about it. It is a very simple concept and you could invent your own scheme by drawing the three faces on card and collecting pictures to put beneath them. Even more basic would be to develop a non-verbal approach which involved nodding or shaking the head or frowning by way of responses.

In many ways the most important sense for those with the greatest communication difficulties is touch. Many people use touch to 'feel out a situation' and convey important emotional messages (see also Chapter Nine on non-verbal approaches) and we have to sensitise ourselves until we are on their wavelength. But touch also gives us special opportunities for sensory activity. There are a number of reports from supporters of innovative approaches to supplying a need through this sense. Sue West noticed how her father became absorbed in coiling the strap of a handbag, so she made him a book, each page consisting of a white card with different textures and colours attached by thread. She went on to make what she called 'fiddlers', a more elaborate play item. She drilled holes in a wooden board and threaded it with colourful pipe-cleaners and laces; he would take this apart and re-assemble it with apparent concentration and satisfaction.

Similar items are actually marketed in the USA under the title 'Twiddlemuffs'. There is a variety of designs available and they are washable. They are described as a 'therapeutic product providing comfort, warmth and movement for those with dementia-related conditions'.

I think the exploration of objects is a significant sensory activity. I have brought stones, shells, small sculptures, woollen and cloth samples and all manner of boxes and bags containing such items to individuals in their own homes and in other environments. I have usually found them to awaken interest. They can be touched, smelt, shaken and tasted as well as inspected visually; the only problems occur when they are so sharp that someone might cut themselves on them or so small that they could be put in the mouth and swallowed. It is frequently the case that the person wants to keep an item for future enjoyment.

Part Two *Other Voices*

Kate Grillet comments on this aspect of communication in relation to Christophe:

> Sensory things were especially important as his verbal language faded: smells of plants, sounds of birds, airplanes passing, hubbub of people, singing, familiar music playing, delicious pureed dishes, which I made every day.

Laurel Rust is a social worker who befriended Amy on a long-stay ward:

> Amy keeps carefully rolled up pieces of paper in her stuffed purse. They are neatly tied up with shreds of toilet paper. Often she has one in her hand. She calls them her 'little

ones'. She keeps them under her pillow, in her drawer, in her bed, until the housekeeper comes through and cleans things up, throws the little ones away and rearranges everything according to institutional order.

One day I made a little one and handed it to her. 'Here's another little one' I said.

'Well, my my,' she said, 'you certainly cracked me.' She laughed and made a face. 'You certainly saw into that one, you blew the whistle on that little story.'

We have met Claire Craig, the occupational therapist, before. Here she is working in a hospital environment, attempting to give significant experiences to individuals through the senses:

Hilda has been in hospital for over ten years now. The ward is her home. She stays in bed for most of the day because of her physical needs. Her limbs are contracted and she spends much time with her hands under her chin. Hilda's sight is poor and she doesn't speak but she makes vocal sounds. From a distance it reminds me of singing.

I enter the bay where she lies, plug in the cassette recorder and begin to play the gentle music. Then, removing the high white bumper sides, I sit down on the bed next to her.

I am wearing a familiar scent and I take her hands in mine, introducing myself and watching for a response. It is a ritual that I have followed many times. Hilda makes positive vocal sounds and for a time I sit so she can get used to the fact that she is no longer alone. Each tiny movement she makes, I mirror, offering reassurance, just enjoying her presence. Then, reaching down I take the first object out of the bag. A fresh sprig of lavender. At first there is no visible response. Five minutes, ten minutes pass, then almost imperceptibly I watch her take it in her hand and lift it to her nose, smelling, touching, sensing the texture. She laughs and I take the second item from the bag. A feather. Again she takes it lifting it, sensing it, touching it, feeling it. I place a little glue on the board. She touches its tackiness. She is smiling now and making eye contact. I tell her how we are going to make this into a sensory collage for her room and the feather floats down onto the surface of the board. I take her hand and we pat it into place together. She pauses and then grabs the feather in her hand pushing it to the top corner and letting it rest there. I smile and tell her it looks much better where she has placed it.

Twenty minutes pass, taking objects, feeling them, sensing them, dropping them onto the board. At times she initiates the movement, and I follow. I am aware that she is becoming tired. I play the tape again and I sit for a moment holding her hand, thanking her for her time and telling her that I will return the next day when we can mount the collage on the wardrobe door. As I leave the ward I hear her voice, singing.

End Note

In our ordinary lives we tend to undervalue the part played by our senses. In dementia they tend to assume even greater significance in communication and relationship. We need to provide increasing opportunities for people to experience through them. One lady, appreciating trees, said:

I think they're just fascinating. I've been mesmerised with them ever since we moved here.

CHAPTER THIRTEEN Keeping in Touch

Part One

In earlier chapters we looked at how the onset of dementia throws up challenges to both the person and their supporters, and how treating this situation as an opportunity rather than a defeat can bring benefits to all. This chapter moves the story on into what is sometimes called 'Advanced Dementia'. The message is the same, though the challenges and opportunities may be different and more intense.

One change which may have to be accommodated is a lack of mobility on the part of the person, so relationships will tend to be confined spatially and revolve around the numerous physical tasks which have to be performed. Dependence becomes an issue here, and possibilities for providing choice and initiative are reduced. This would, of course, be the same for anyone confined to bed or a wheelchair, but in this case there may also be the occurrence of loss of verbal fluency, which places an added responsibility on us to find new ways to stimulate responses and interpret signs.

The chapter on non-verbal communication provides guidance here, and the one on sensual approaches may also prove helpful. It is undeniable, however, that for some people extending one's range in these ways can prove daunting, whereas others may display a natural facility in developing such approaches. What is certain is that a loving relationship can carry you through most things you will encounter.

I am devoting the rest of this chapter to two brief descriptions of meetings with people which occurred during a project set up to explore ways of getting in contact with people with profound communication difficulties. I had read about the principles of 'Coma Work', and I wanted to try out the fundamental techniques of eye contact, touch, body language, tone of voice and singing with people who were at that stage in their lives when there might be some applicability. On this journey I was accompanied by a video-maker and a sound-recordist. I did not know either of the people with dementia that I worked with beforehand, which had its advantages and disadvantages: there was no relationship to build on, but there were no preconceptions to jettison. Both sets of interactions proved to our satisfaction that communication was possible and that it could throw a lifeline to the individuals concerned.

PEGGY

Peggy was very variable in her actions and reactions. Generally, it took quite a long time for her to begin to respond. We met in her room, and she sat in a chair, as did I. In the first session she seemed wary and ambivalent, until somehow I was able to anticipate and match, almost exactly in time, an extended and complex vocalisation she made. That was the turning-point: she began to make eye-contact and to hold my hand, instead of reacting passively or avoiding my attempts to make physical contact with her. Following this, I hummed a tune to her and she looked directly at me throughout.

The next session was cut short because she seemed unwell and not to welcome my presence. The third session, which lasted 23 minutes, had a clear overall structure. For the first ten minutes she was turned away from me and did not interact overtly. However, after this time she turned her body towards me and there followed eight minutes of intense interaction: she made eye contact, smiled, laughed and spoke fluently (though I could not understand the words). She looked around her room, especially in the direction of family photographs on the wall. I played her the tune Edelweiss on a music-box; she demonstrated pleasure by nodding and smiling and uttering word-like sounds (I made out 'yes' as one of them) clearly in relation to it. Then she turned away and appeared to resume the state she had been in earlier.

The fourth session was special in a different way. It took her 25 minutes to become fully aware of my presence and availability to her, but once she did begin to interact her mood seemed very different from on other occasions. Her face had a fierce expression, and she took both my hands in hers and rubbed them, manipulated them violently, and dug her nails into them for around 17 minutes, before releasing them and turning away again. This session reminded me of the great variety of emotions that people need to express.

NANCY

She was physically frail, in a bed with high safety rails, and was being fed by a nasogastric tube. I visited her on several occasions only to find her asleep.

Our first encounter when I found her awake was very active. As I approached her she made eye-contact immediately, and smiled and laughed a number of times. She responded positively to my holding her hand by reciprocating my grip. Although she made many vocal sounds, it was only on re-hearing the high quality recordings that I realised how distinctive they were. The actual words were indistinct but utterances were formed, rhythmical, and appeared to be in response to my remarks, and also matched the smiling and laughing that occurred.

The second session was shorter and less distinctive, but the third was extended (44 minutes), intense, and of a very different character from the first. There was no smiling or laughing, but Nancy maintained eye contact and held my hand tightly. After 23 minutes of interacting I suggested she might be getting tired and began to initiate a departure. After getting as far as standing up and moving my stool, I sat down again because of the urgency of her eye-contact, and an utterance which sounded very like 'I don't want you to go'. Nancy proceeded, with great effort, to manoeuvre her right hand out from under her body so that she could hold both of my hands with both of hers. The session continued for another 19 minutes at Nancy's insistence, before she had a coughing fit and nursing staff had to be brought in. This was an abrupt and distressing ending to the interaction. I am sure that the choking was caused by the length of the session, but I had been responding to self-evident need. I came away with a new understanding of the significance of human contact for individuals even close to the end of their lives (Nancy died less than a month later).

Part Two *Other Voices*

Frena Gray Davidson has the following observation about people who seem to be unconnected to events around them:

> This sense of interior preoccupation is often found in the later stages of Alzheimer's. They give the impression not of being the living dead, but of being the absorbed absentee off away doing other things. It never seems to be a distressed state, always one of quiet absorption. Some people in such states have even been taken to hospital... only to be sent home diagnosed as being in an altered state.

Rosemary Clarke, who supported her mother over a long period, has written about using the Coma technique:

> From the vantage point of several months since first using just the basics of Coma work with my mother, it is blindingly obvious. Before that I had been labouring unsuccessfully to communicate to my mother. Now I am seeking to help her to communicate outwards: to whom-

ever/whatever. The fact that she cannot speak (to all intents and purposes) merely means that she is largely post-verbal. She has, it turns out when I really pay attention, several ways of expressing herself. And the miracle is that in so doing she once again engages with me, sometimes very directly and purposefully.

In the event, so much else has happened which I thought would never happen again. Although I have written mostly in measured, descriptive language, my experience has been at times sublime and I believe for her empowering. We can communicate without words at least to an acceptable degree, and sometimes in a way that is quite beautiful, even awesome, allowing great intimacy.

In the field of communication with people like my mother at this point in her life, I look forward to the time when it is the norm for all carers, professional and family, automatically to assume that the person *does* have things to 'say' and that it is up to us to find ways of 'hearing'.

My experience with my mother in these last few months has been infinitely precious and enriching for me, and I commend this approach to others who would like to both give and gain deep satisfaction in their contact with those with dementia who are, largely, beyond words.

End Note

Probably the greatest challenge dementia presents is communicating with those who have lost the power of speech. Nevertheless, if we are prepared to learn new skills and to persevere, the rewards are there, and they are of a unique and memorable nature. In the following extract from a longer sequence I have tried to give expression to this:

Your body speaks the lines
your mouth can no longer utter
and I am here to learn them.

Each posture, every gesture,
that glint in the eye, cry, turn down
of the mouth, pressure of the fingertips –

are not to be taken in isolation,
but make up a composite
of who you were and are.

CHAPTER FOURTEEN **Being Creative**

Part One

If we are looking for areas in which people with dementia might excel, then we may have found one in the arts. Let's think first about childhood – not because people with the condition have reverted, but because of one special characteristic they share with children, and that is an innocence of appreciation. Of course children have never known anything else, but perhaps because of living in the moment (see Chapter Sixteen for more about this) things come up fresh for people, a sense of wonder is easier to come by.

The move from intellect to emotion and the emphasis on feeling over reasoning in the arts may also make creativity especially appealing.

Then there is the fact that the arts involve activity. Yes, there is the matter of appreciation, being part of an audience, which is more passive, but fundamentally they are about doing, being involved in something, whether or not there is an end product. And I hardly need emphasize that many older people suffer from a chronic lack of activity.

The arts are also about communication, getting a message across in a vivid and unusual way. And many art forms (music, painting, dance, sculpture, for example) don't involve words, which provides an outlet for those for whom the verbal causes problems.

There is also the matter of beauty – the marriage of a message and the craft to express it can result in an object which can be admired for its aesthetic qualities.

Lastly there is what we call the therapeutic element. Sometimes this can involve specially trained experts. But I am thinking of a more generalised quality: the person has feelings bottled up, and the creative activity encourages release. This can increase the experience of wellbeing in the short term and may have longer effects too.

So in all these ways the arts offer people with dementia special opportunities to make a contribution, and offer those of us in a supporting role special opportunities to get alongside them. What do people themselves have to say about this?

One day I was sharing some postcards of artworks she

loved with a lady and she turned to me and with a sense of urgency said, 'The arts is all that's left. Give them us!'

*

Claire Craig, the occupational therapist, had been engaging with a lady on a craft activity when she said:

> 'We have been on a wonderful journey, you and I. What fun we've had, laughing and singing. Holding a rainbow in our hands.'

*

Katie Clark works for the Reader Organisation and reads poetry with people. One man commented:

> 'It moves you. I mean, it hits you inside where it meets you and means something.'

Some years ago I was making a radio programme to show how I helped people with dementia to write poems. I approached a feisty man from Glasgow, Ian McQueen, to take part. He declined in forceful terms. 'I hated poetry at school,' he said. 'It was rubbish.' But I prevailed, by explaining that all he needed to do was talk, I would record his words, and if I could I'd shape poems from them. By the end of the sixth session, not only had Ian clearly enjoyed himself hugely, but we had made seven or eight poems. I asked him what he thought of poetry now. He said, 'Poetry is essence of essences... What matters to me is the **me-ness** of it.' (Four of Ian's poems are in the book *Dementia Diary* – see the back of this book.)

I don't want to give the impression that helping people to be creative is only a role for the artistically trained, for those 'in the know'. It is definitely for everyone, and provides opportunities for a special sharing to take place in which supporters too can benefit hugely.

The growth of the 'Singing For the Brain' movement in the UK over recent years attests to the appeal of communal musical activity: it taps into the latent memories of people and is stimulating socially.

Painting and crafts come a close second to music in popularity, mainly because there is such variety under this banner, from sketching to collage, from mandalas to macramé. There are many 'how to' books on the market, and one very special one by Sarah Zoutewelle-Morris (details at the back of this book).

Speaking of books, there is a set of picture books created specifically for people with dementia called *Pictures to Share*. They were designed and marketed by the daughter of someone who loved books but could no longer read. As the title of the series indicates, they are really good for looking at and discussing together.

We must not forget the appreciation side of creativity: going to concerts, galleries, theatres etc. I have found that sometimes people's response to works of art has actually been enhanced by the condition: they are more insightful and enthusiastic than they were before. This has certainly been a finding of the Artz for Alzheimer's movement in

America; their practice of taking groups of people to galleries has proved wildly successful, and is spreading throughout the world, and they are also experimenting with hiring cinemas for special showings.

Part Two *Other Voices*

Agnes Houston is a younger woman who, in the following passage, reflects both on the way dementia has freed her up for new experiences, and also recognizes that the arts may fulfil a new need that she has developed:

> I'm not saying that dementia's not serious. But I'm going to say that it's a licence in a way, a licence to be free, to be me. I think when I got the diagnosis I got permission to be more relaxed into this person and accept her.
>
> I wanted to find out if I was artistic. Creativity's an aspect I want to explore. Being able to feel out of the box is what I'm picking up. It will happen. It's a bit like waiting on Christmas. You know it's coming but as a child you don't exactly know when. It's a nice feeling.

Listening to music can be a consoling experience, as Cary Smith Henderson eloquently shows in this passage:

> I've always loved music very very deeply and I find this a solace... I've whiled away many many hours listening to music and feel that I'm doing something that I just love to do. I can't make music anymore, but I can certainly use it for my own intentions – which are just to be beautiful.

Dance, both the expressive and social kinds, is another

important area for communication, and Heather Hill, a dance therapist in Australia, explains why:

> Movement and dance involve the whole body – obviously as human beings we are embodied, which means that we experience the world and our being in our bodies, and express ourselves and communicate with others through our bodies. We tend to forget this and place total emphasis on our minds as the source of self and of our personhood. No wonder dementia, which attacks the mind, is so frightening. However, even when our mind is fully functioning, our experience of and interaction with the world comes through the body... In the dance, an experience which is not dependent on verbal skills, the person is more able to connect with other people. We are also more able to connect with them.

Oliver Sacks, the neurologist, commented on the process of taking groups of people to look at pictures in a gallery:

> Certainly it's not just a visual experience – it's an emotional one. In an informal way I have often seen quite demented patients recognise and respond vividly to paintings and delight in painting at a time when they are scarcely responsive to words and disoriented out of it. I think that recognition of visual art can be very deep.

End Note

The arts may have something special to offer people who are cognitively challenged: a sense of wonder, an outlet for feelings, meaningful activity, a medium of communication, an appeal to the aesthetic sense, and a sense of release. There is great variety – you just need a series of try-outs to see what suits the person. There are opportunities for appreciation as well as practical activity. One man in a poem put things in his own way:

> to see what is beautiful
> to hear what is beautiful
> they don't know what is beautiful...
>
> we see it very rarely
> but the difference is
> we are trying to see!

CHAPTER FIFTEEN **Cultivating Playfulness**

Part One

I can hear my readers muttering at this point: 'Playful? But dementia's no joke!' And you are of course right. But I want to suggest to you that taking a lighter approach to problems can often ease the burden for all concerned.

In adopting this approach I am aware of running counter to some quite strong currents in society. One attitude which prevails is that play is for children, and something that we are expected to grow out of. At school we imbibe the principle that work is what life is about, and play is hived off into organized games. Even these are given a serious component when they become competitive. Also, the intellectual bias of our educational system excludes play as a frivolous irrelevance, only to be indulged in as spare-time hobbies. Any advocacy of play for older adults is liable to be viewed with suspicion, and perhaps subject to comments about 'second childhood'.

But we all have a need not to take ourselves too seriously. Think of the number of times in your life when laughter took the tension out of a situation, or suddenly transformed your understanding of an issue. In certain contexts, when practised consistently, playfulness can turn a chore into a pleasure.

Can it do more? Charlie Chaplin said, 'to truly laugh you must take your pain and play with it.' If we apply this to dementia, is it possible that approaching the condition in a spirit of playfulness can actually make it more bearable, both for the person and their supporters? I believe it can.

Let me give an example from my own experience. I have been developing an activity for groups of people based on improvised drama games that I call 'Funshops'. I lead the activity, but many of the ideas come from the participants. People benefit from being freed up to say and do things spontaneously. The sessions also provide a respite for individuals from the changes that may be occurring in their perceptions and relationships. Furthermore, there is a sense of community engendered, and significant bondings can occur. These characteristics are illustrated by the following story:

A man (let's call him Albert) in one of the groups on the

first occasion showed great reluctance to attend, but he had been sent there by his wife. He was made welcome and encouraged to become involved. I found out that he had been an amateur artist, so at the second meeting of the group I thought up a special sketch for us to do together. I put him in charge of the improvisation: he was an artist and I was the client who had commissioned him to paint my portrait. As my demands as to how the picture was to be painted grew ever more absurd Albert kept a straight face. Eventually he turned to the rest of the group and said quite simply 'I resign.' Everyone fell about laughing. He had played the role perfectly: in particular his timing was impeccable. At the third, Funshop Albert told everyone that his attitude to his condition had completely changed as a result of attending the sessions. He no longer wished to hide because of his dementia but was going out to meet people and having fun.

In the chapter on managing, I referred to the possible power differential between a person with the condition and those around them. We have to be aware of this in relation to playfulness. Whilst turning a difficult situation into a joke can bring positive benefits, there is a danger of this being interpreted as ridiculing a person's disability (this is what Kitwood called 'mockery'). There must be a strong and mutual respect in the relationship for this kind of approach to work.

Playfulness without words, I believe, is just as important as where the verbal is involved. On many occasions I have been attempting communication with someone whose verbal ability is severely restricted and I have sensed a laugh welling up in the other person which I can match at the moment it breaks out. And even where that has not occurred, though I may not know what has occasioned a laugh, I find I can join in. This is because, as is so often stated, laughter is infectious. So my advice is, wherever possible, let's start an epidemic!

Part Two *Other Voices*

The writer Elizabeth Cohen has put the case for humour most succinctly:

> I think that a sense of humour must be hidden in a box very deep in the brain, where diseases have to search for it. Maybe this is an evolutionary tactic, to keep people going.

We have met Richard Taylor, a person with dementia, in other chapters. Here he is on the importance of humour:

> Laughing is a common denominator of our humanity. Laughter, intense laughing, is what separates humans from all other forms of life on our planet. Animals can be happy, but they cannot laugh out loud, laugh until they cry or until their sides hurt. People living with dementia can laugh that hard. Unfortunately they seldom do. We should share, encourage, and point out all moments of joy and glee to one another, especially to people living with dementia whose lives are too much defined by sadness. Laughter can reinforce the joy, the purposefulness, the connectedness

of all human beings – if only we can see the forest of humanity instead of the trees of dementia.

Agnes Houston, whom we have already encountered in the previous chapter, is someone who plays an important role in a very active organization, The Scottish Dementia Working Group:

I didn't think I had a sense of humour. I was too busy being serious. Then when I got dementia I was having to focus on myself for the first time in a long time. Suddenly I had to look at myself to see what I could put in place, who was this different Agnes? The Group started talking about humour. Then it was fed back to me that I do have a sense of humour, so do my brothers. Then I started using humour in a lot of things. I can see the fun in a situation, and I can feel myself smiling internally, then it comes into my face. I can find fun in a lot of situations that can be quite serious, like everybody else is losing their cool, and I can feel a bit of fun and bring it in, and before you know it people are beginning to be a bit more lighthearted. It takes the sting out of a lot of sore situations. There's a lot of humour in the SDWG and it's that type of humour. When you're sitting there they might bring up quite a sad situation and then you might get David spilling it into looking at it from a different angle. I realise I had that there all the time.

Kim Zabbia lets us in on one of her playful strategies in relation to her mother:

My son Ricky gave me a sweatshirt for Christmas. On

the front it said 'I remembered'. On the back it said 'I forgot. Al took it.' Who is Al? Al is Mrs Zheimer's son, Al Zheimer. I know it's corny, but it beats dwelling on the sad side of the story.

End Note

Playfulness is one of the ways of being creative in our approach to relationships. We all know people who can help us to laugh at life's little tribulations, and some of its bigger ones as well, and we value them for it. You can be such a person in regard to someone with the condition. It is a sign of trust and empathy if you can encourage a mirthful outlook. One man with dementia said to me:

> I never felt so well – it's the laughter, it keeps me young, it beats all the drugs.

CHAPTER SIXTEEN **Living in the Moment**

Part One

Sandy had always seemed to me rather a depressed person, and I thought this state of mind might well have contributed in some way to his dementia. One day I heard him speaking to the head of the unit. 'What pain ever goes?' he reflected. On another occasion he said to me, 'I'm all muddled up. I'm useless. I'm nearly crying.' I tried to reassure him, 'You're a really nice man, Sandy,' I said. 'Nice man's not enough on its own. Far better to be nice man *and* what you've got,' he replied.

The following day Sandy greeted me with handshakes and smiles. I sensed a complete change of mood in him. The unit was built on a courtyard system with a garden in the middle. He set off along the corridor which would eventually bring him back to where I was standing. Suddenly he was running and jumping as he completed the circuit, and singing at the top of his voice. As he passed me he shouted, 'It's time to do some work. To work and sing.' He seemed overflowing with energy and happiness.

When he came round for the second time Sandy paused and said to me, 'Don't stop being beyond us, because that's what we need.' He took my hand and we set off together. I didn't know the words or the music, but I followed his lead. We hopped and skipped, and sang all the way round the square.

Then Sandy paused and turned to me. 'What are we doing here?' he asked. 'I have no idea,' I answered, 'but does it matter?' 'Why are we doing this?' was his follow-up question. 'Because we want to,' I replied. He seemed perfectly satisfied by this, and we both roared with laughter and embraced. Then he disengaged his hand and danced on. He kept this high energy activity up for a further twenty minutes before, apparently exhausted, coming for his tea.

This was an astonishing episode, because of its intensity and its duration, but also because of its unpredictability. It could not have been anticipated, and I am not aware of its causation. It proceeded spontaneously and came from the person. For that period of time Sandy seemed to be living fully and wholly in the moment.

This raises the question of whether people with dementia have a capacity which the rest of us may only strive for: that of being able to exist in the present, without hankering after past or future. It is certainly something that individuals with the condition are telling us. Laura Smith says, 'Most of the time I live in the space I can see and the time called now.' And John Zeisel lists this as one of 'The Gifts of Alzheimer's' (see Chapter 2).

Maybe this is one of the aspects of dementia which we should be marking up as a positive? In which case surely we should be attempting to foster opportunities for people to experience what might be called 'nowness' to make their lives as meaningful and pleasurable as possible? And by doing so could we also, by a process of osmosis, be enriching the lives of all who come into contact with them, including ourselves?

Part Two *Other Voices*

John Zeisel, the American writer and activist whom we have already met in these pages, has this to say about time:

> People living with Alzheimer's tend more and more to experience a point rather than a line of time. Someone might talk about a long-dead relative as if he were just about to arrive for a visit. Or a daughter of sixty is seen as a sister of thirty. It is as if past experience and the future have drawn together with the present as one; much like

how our unconscious minds combine several dimensions of time and place when we dream. The present moment represents all moments.

Laurel Rust, whom we met in Chapter Twelve, in her role as a social worker in America, describes her relationship with Amy in the following terms:

Amy and I have developed an intimacy that is hard to describe, an intimacy that makes me think of companionship differently because Amy does not know my name and has never asked. We sit and simply take up talking whenever and wherever we are. Talking with Amy who 'exhibits no orientation to reality' is a wonderful experience in which we are always in the present, and the present could be anything we choose to create between us.

Judith Maizels describes the change in attitude which occurred visiting her mother in a care facility when she realised the potential for growth that it offered:

At first I used to call my journey in the lift up to the 'Reminiscence Community' as taking me 'halfway to Hell', but now I feel it is really 'halfway to Heaven'. As I travel upwards in the lift I silently pray for light, love and healing for all. When the door opens, I take a deep breath, and step forward through a doorway into a different world. Here time itself takes on a different dimension. Time does not pass faster or more slowly than in the outer world; instead, it takes on a transcendent quality. My experience of time is transformed, reflecting the fact that the emotional intensity of each moment seems to become vividly heightened.

In this last extract an anonymous family carer reflects on what her mother has taught her:

> Mom and I were taking a walk, and as hard as I tried to be attentive my mind was on my own problems. I was thinking about work, a problem in my marriage, and some financial decisions. My mother suddenly said, 'Look at that!' I looked up towards a group of trees and could see nothing. She said 'Look at that beautiful bird.' I still couldn't see it. Finally, as I scanned the limbs, it was there.
>
> The incident made me reflect on my mother's world and my own. Now, she always finds the beautiful birds in the tree, or smells the scent of flowers in the air, and hears music in the distance. I had shut all these out. Her Alzheimer's had somehow put her back in touch with nature and the spiritual side of her life. I had perfect cognition, but I wasn't seeing any of the world around me. Maybe there were still some things I could learn from her.

End Note

People with dementia may experience a different time-scale from the rest of us. If so, we should we respect this, and learn to use it for their, and our, benefit. I have tried to encapsulate the message of this chapter in the following haiku:

> This gift I bring you,
> please handle it carefully:
> it is the present.

CHAPTER SEVENTEEN **A Home from Home**

Part One

My first ten years with people with dementia were spent exclusively in care homes, and I have worked in many since. So I think I may have earned the right to say that in what follows I am speaking from experience. In design, facilities, staffing, leadership and atmosphere they differ widely. Put this together with the uniqueness of each individual with the condition, and you will appreciate the dilemma I face in trying to generalise. Nevertheless, there are a number of things I feel I can say.

One is that for some people the transition from their own home is difficult, and may be resisted for a long time. They inevitably miss their own surroundings, where they can practise their long-established routines without interruption. Some individuals are fiercely independent, and this is a good quality which they should surely be encouraged to maintain.

The man who had recently been admitted and bitterly complained that 'the cups of tea here all end half-way up' probably fell into this category. He told me, 'I've been sent here on a golfing holiday, and they haven't even got a course.' This may have indicated that he wasn't yet ready to accept his situation. He clearly appreciated the opportunity to 'sound off' to someone who wasn't in authority. Another man refused to have conversations with me 'because you don't have a key to the door,' responding strongly to the fact that he was living on a locked unit.

Some people do not resent confinement but find a communal environment conducive to making new friendships and enjoying activities new and old. They don't regret losing the isolation which was often their lot prior to admission. One woman commented extensively on the deficiencies of the men on the unit, whilst also appreciating their company. She remarked, 'I get on with all these men alright. And if they want to do anything I tell them how: that the best way to get on in life is to agree with me.'

In one home I helped a woman by writing down her thoughts. 'My memory, it slims away,' was one of the things she said, already quoted in Chapter Seven. Her husband seemed very appreciative of what I was doing for his wife. 'I've got a lot I need to get off my chest. I wonder if you could do this for me?' he asked. We had a number of sessions in which I recorded him and transcribed the tapes later. He talked about what he felt about his wife's condition and her admission to the home. He said he had found this very helpful. Then one day his wife expressed the wish to write something for her husband. We struggled for a couple of hours getting a tribute down on paper. She asked me to give it to him on his next visit. It did not go according to plan. When he saw the piece of writing he would not read it, screwed it up and threw it away. He said he didn't need me to prove to him that his wife was ill. I was surprised by this as he had seemed most sympathetic to the process. Maybe I had caught him on a bad day. But it could be that this story illustrates how distress is often deep-seated in a close relative – sometimes this is about not having come to terms with the changes that have occurred in the loved one. Sometimes it comes from guilt at having not been able to continue looking after them at home.

Perhaps in this situation someone could seek counselling, or the support of family members, or of those in a similar situation. I don't wish to underestimate the degree of adjustment involved in allowing others to take over the care you have been delivering, often for a long time.

Some family members have found it really helpful to immerse themselves in the life of the home, not just being with their relative for regular periods, but interacting with others with dementia, staff and supporters. In other words, they consider the home as a small community, with all the possibilities for developing relationships, sharing in activities, and being of service that that implies.

It is sometimes remarked that staff only seem to see the person as they are now, without taking into account how they were earlier in their lives. It must be very easy, caught up in a busy schedule, to become absorbed in practical tasks, but a supporter can help by taking in photographs, family videos and stories. A life history book in pictorial form, with easy-to-read captions, can prove invaluable as a reminder of a person's past and became a real focus for discussion. The same approach becomes vital when someone enters hospital for a period, and there is less time available and often less continuity in staff coverage.

The whole business of compiling a life book can be an enjoyable collaborative activity. Someone described the process in the following words: 'You climb up the family tree and look at the vista from there.'

Part Two *Other Voices*

Rebecca Ley pays tribute to the staff in the home where her father lives, and the qualities they display in carrying out ordinary tasks:

> Fear has a way of sucking the joy out of life's smaller pleasures – cups of tea, slices of cake, good songs on the radio, juicy gossip, and some carers are really skilled at reclaiming it. Composure is also important. When someone is slowly and inexorably losing control of their bladder and bowels, with all the attendant accidents and embarrassment, a certain sang-froid is welcome.
>
> I've also noticed that Dad's best carers demonstrate great flexibility. They will pick up whatever scraps of dialogue he throws out and spin them out into something like a conversation. They are pleased by his compliments, interested in his odd declarations.
>
> They are also tactile. They don't shy away from his hugs or flinch when he wants to stroke their faces. They don't deprive him of that fundamental human need to touch someone else, and in that way they dignify him.

And here is the second part of the story told by Laura Beck which began in the chapter on fear. There, if you recall, she found her father's conduct alienating, and wished herself away from the home in which she was visiting him:

> So I went in, sat beside him, and took his hand while he sang. We connected with our eyes – eye contact was something I hadn't gotten from him in a very long time. I began to envy him as I watched him dance between the worlds. He was exploring places I couldn't begin to go...
>
> I found I felt honoured to share that moment with him, to play a part in his unhurried dance out of this world; to have witnessed his last steps a few months ago, and to have heard him utter my name for the last time almost three years previously.
>
> Watching him I did not see him as the victim of a debilitating disease, but rather as an inspired messenger. He was entirely in the moment – full of unfettered playfulness. How long had it been since I'd stopped to celebrate a moment so exuberantly?
>
> So I joined in and chanted with him... This was one of the most intense and delightful connections I had ever had in the history of my relationship with my father. His eyes met mine for the first time in years. Deeply moved, I thanked him for the wisdom he had offered me – a reminder to savour the precious gift of every moment. And I realized... had I succumbed to my fear I would have missed it all.

I am sure I am not alone in seeing links in this extract, not just to the fear chapter, but to the non-verbal, playfulness and living in the moment ones as well.

End Note

Transitions are difficult for everyone concerned. Once a person is settled in the new environment we need to be prepared for fresh relationships and ways of making a contribution. But above all, we must maintain our constancy of concern for the loved one. Here is a daughter showing real understanding of the situation her father finds himself in:

> Some people tell my father he should not visit my mother in the nursing home so often and that he should take up other activities. He does do other things, but visiting my mother is what he needs to do.

CHAPTER EIGHTEEN **A Good Sunset**

Part One

One day I was in a lounge in a care home and I heard a lady singing a sad song in the corner of the room. When I got up close these are some of her words:

> O World
> I don't know what to do
> I want to see my sunset
> I want it as it was promised
> I'm waiting for the hour
> I want to see my sunset good

There are many griefs associated with dementia. Some belong to the person. Some are likely to be experienced by those around them. And some can be felt in common.

The griefs of the person, particularly one with increasing

communication problems, may be difficult to identify and therefore to address. The same is true of those with the condition who may be experiencing physical pain. Whether the pain is in the mind or the body or both, if they have lost the ability to tell you about it, there can be no substitute for attempting to understand the facial expressions and physical gestures unique to that person. It involves concentrated effort over a period of time. There is a theory that emotional pain in people with dementia is likely to be general rather than specific, so you may not know exactly what is causing it. In these circumstances all you can do is be there for the person and offer as much comfort as you can. This is one of the most difficult circumstances you have to contend with in relating to someone with the condition.

The griefs that supporters feel can involve the past (how things might have turned out if you had acted differently), the present (how to cope with current problems as they are thrown up), and the future (both in terms of unrealised plans, and of how things may turn out).

Despite the tendency to be overwhelmed by these griefs, you have to find ways of rising above them. The key to this is as fully as possible living life in the moment, as advocated in Chapter Sixteen. In this, hopefully, the person can show you the way. You need first of all to become convinced that changing what is past, or living in the might-have-beens, or imagining the worst of scenarios, are counter-productive. You could drag yourself down, and the person with you. I am convinced that the positives will be there if you look for them.

Where griefs are shared, then the old adage about problems being halved surely still applies. What the person brings to this is the immediacy of their involvement. What you bring is your quality of empathy and your eagerness to learn. It could be a winning combination. Many who have wholeheartedly embraced this collaboration have spoken of the maturing nature of the experience.

As the person nears the end of their life, you would expect to have feelings of imminent loss. There are stories of a new level of intensive identification occurring. In a sense, it has all been leading up to this. Irrespective of any religious belief they may have, some speak of an experience of heightened spirituality.

After a death has occurred, to judge by many personal accounts I have been given, these feelings of closeness are slow to diminish. The impression is of a major human event one has been privileged to be a part of.

Part Two *Other Voices*

John Zeisel (quotes from whom are to be found in the chapters on the nature of dementia, and the moment) makes an important distinction:

> While pain is a given, suffering is optional. My teachers have been husbands and wives, siblings and children, friends and grandchildren who have avoided suffering by

embracing their loved ones as they are; by living in the present moment of Alzheimer's with its humour, pathos, fun and joy as well as pain.

These quotations all come from supporters: Jane, Marsha, Carl and Debbie:

One blessing is that I have gotten through a big part of the grief process. I have now accepted the husband I have today. I have learned to go with his flow whenever possible. This is a wonderful gift. It has taken a few years to reach this point, but it has freed me of the need to control every situation. I often feel as if I divorced the former husband and married a similar man. He looks the same but responds very differently to most parts of our former lifestyle.

*

The last few months of my mother's life were in some ways the best in our relationship. She had been very demanding all of her life, but now she was open in a way she had never been before. We became closer than I imagined we could.

*

I'd had a difficult relationship with my mother. Her dying seemed endless and her existence pointless, and at times I felt as if once again she'd never do what we wanted her to do. I kept asking myself, 'Why doesn't she die?' But after she died I could see that this long dying was a time of healing for both of us. I could hold her hand and sing to her and read psalms, and I think she felt loved as well.

This time with her was a gift, for all its difficulty, and I'm a different person because of it.

*

Not all the changes dementia brings are negative ones. My relationship with my grandma changed – but without dementia I don't feel I would ever have been so close to her or would ever have shared so many special moments.

And lastly from Helen Finch, who has shared her insights a number of times before:

When I came to my mother on the last visit – she wasn't feeling very well, she seemed very stressed – we sat in her room and she clung onto me, put her arm round me, and repeated over and over 'Daddy, Daddy, Daddy!' Now to me that wasn't a bad thing, it was a most wonderful experience. Because knowing a little bit about her past, that, I think, was her way of expressing the fact that I could give her something, and that I was very special to her. It was more touching, more moving, and communicated more, than if she had called me by my real name.

End Note

Grief is an essential part of this condition, as it is of life itself, and of dying. How we cope with it is a matter for individuals, but there are strategies we can develop which can benefit ourselves and others. Sometimes the journey in retrospect assumes a new perspective. Betsy Peterson found that for herself:

I would never have believed this could be true, but sometimes I miss the intensity of the caregiving years. It was a time of living close to the core of life.

CHAPTER NINETEEN **Making Preparations**

Most of us would not naturally and comfortably choose to contemplate the prospect of being diagnosed with the condition to which this book has been devoted. Difficult emotions might be aroused by doing so. We may consider that there is no point in distressing ourselves by speculating in this manner. Nevertheless it must have crossed our minds at some time or another, particularly if we are close to someone going through the experience: could it be me next? And, of course, statistically speaking, many of us will develop dementia. It seemed important, therefore, to devote this final chapter to a consideration of this possibility.

In terms of the image that gave its title to the 1997 Alzheimer's Disease International Conference held in Helsinki, many of us, readers of and contributors to this volume, will be singled out to be struck by the arrow of 'The Blind Hunter'. This emphasizes the apparently random nature of its occurrence.

So, assume that you will be one of those people in the future, what can you do in advance to prepare for that eventuality? One thing would be to take legal advice and make provision in the form of directives. The various Alzheimer's Societies and their local branches can certainly help here too. But what other planning can you do?

I suggest you put all other concerns aside for an hour and tackle the questions at the end of the chapter. Then look at the answers you have assembled. If you were no longer in a position to tell someone any of these things, would the information you have provided be a help to them? Would there be other things you would want them to know? Further lists could be about music, colours, clothes, scents, hobbies, films, TV programmes... Our lives are complex, and we are all individuals, and it is impossible in a series of questions to cover everyone's priorities.

You may feel that a list like this is too simplistic and you would prefer to take more time over the exercise and go into greater detail. Here are three suggestions for more active preparation:

- Make a 30-minute tape telling people what you most want them to know about you. This could include answers to the list of questions and many other things.
- Make another tape of 30 minutes of music which are of special significance to you, and which would bear repetition over the months and years ahead.
- Arrange a photograph album of the people and places in your life which were and are of most importance to you and which can be used as prompts for your memory.

These could be of value to anyone as grounding activities, reminders to the self of the significance of person-centredness. They help us to evaluate our concerns and to take stock of our lives.

Those who are singled out are embarking on a voyage within life into a mysterious future. Surely we should consider taking these elementary steps to provide for our needs? The Ancient Egyptians used to place a little food and drink and loved objects beside the bodies of their dead when they were entombed. These were the preparations they made on behalf of those who were setting out on a long journey.

PLANNING STRATEGY

- If you were to lose all other possessions in a fire in your home, which two or three small objects would you save and why are they most important to you?
- If you had had a bad day, what would be the single thing that would most console you?
- You are about to set out on a long journey from which you may not return. Who are the persons closest to you? Write each of them a postcard-length message saying what you value about them.
- Make a list of the physical comforts which mean most to you.
- What activity helps you to start the day positively?
- Describe two or three paintings or photographs which you would like to have close to you.
- Name two or three pieces of writing (poetry or prose) which you feel you would never tire of reading.
- Make up a day's menus consisting of your favourite foods and drinks.

- Describe any particular fears or dislikes that you have.
- Name and describe some special places in your life.

POSTSCRIPT

So we have come to the end of this book, and I am only too conscious of the things I have not said, and those I might have said better.

When you are dealing with a condition which raises so many profound questions about what it means to be human it is inevitable that any text remains provisional and unsatisfactory.

But I remain passionately convinced of the following:

1. that we cannot wait for medical science to provide the big answers (maybe they will never deliver the goods!) but must act in small ways to transform all our lives in the present;

2. that concentrating on exploring ways to communicate with and relate to people is the way forward and will lead to fresh insights;

3. that the advances we will make in this area will benefit both those with the condition and those who support them – indeed have the capacity to change much of Dementia Negative into Dementia Positive.

If you have some experiences of this kind that you would be happy to share, please email me at:

johnkillick@dementiapositive.co.uk

Oh, I almost forgot – I wonder if you have looked back at that riddle by Oliver Sacks with which I began Chapter

Two? Do you see anything more in it now than you did first time round?

And perhaps you would like to look at it alongside this quotation (my last, I promise you!) from Christine Bryden:

> I believe that people with dementia are making an important journey from cognition, through emotion, into spirit. I've begun to realise what really remains throughout this journey is what is really important, and what disappears is what is not important. I think that if society could appreciate this, then people with dementia would be treasured and respected.

WHERE THE QUOTES COME FROM

In case you want to follow any of them up, and also by way of acknowledgement to all the authors and sources involved.

Chapter One

The book by Richard Cheston and Michael Bender is called *Understanding Dementia: The Man With Worried Eyes* and was published by Jessica Kingsley in 1999. Peter Whitehouse's book (co-written with Danny George) came from St Martin's Press in 2008 and is titled *The Myth of Alzheimer's: What you aren't being told about today's most dreaded diagnosis.*

Richard Taylor's quote comes from his book *Alzheimer's From the Inside Out*, published by Health Professions Press Inc. in 2007.

Christine Bryden's quote comes from her 1997 book *Who Will I Be When I Die?* published by Harper Collins, and now available from Jessica Kingsley Publications.

Bob Fay wrote this in an article entitled *What a Very Unfriendly word 'dementia' is* in the Alzheimer's Society Newsletter in December 2003.

Joanne Koenig Coste's book *Learning to Speak Alzheimer's* was published by Houghton Mifflin in 2004.

Chapter Two

The Oliver Sacks quote comes from a radio broadcast, and is quoted with his permission.

Tom Kitwood's list of examples of 'malignant social psychology' can be found in his book *Dementia Reconsidered: the person comes first* published by Open University Press in 1997.

Joanne Koenig Coste: see Chapter One.

I'm Still Here by John Zeisel was published by Penguin in the USA in 2009. It has been brought out in the UK by Piatkus.

Richard Taylor: see Chapter One.

Chapter Three

Deborah Everett's book from which the quote comes is *Forget-Me-Not: The Spiritual Care of People with Alzheimer's* published in 1996 by Inkwell Press, Edmonton, Canada.

The story by Laura Beck comes from a book by G Allen Power *Dementia Beyond Drugs: Changing the Culture of Care* published by Health Professions Press.

The Prophet is available in a variety of editions.

Chapter Four

Details of K H Zabbia's book can be found under notes to Chapter Fifteen.

Scar Tissue by Michael Ignatieff was published by Vintage in 1994.

James McKillop's contribution forms part of a chapter entitled 'Did Research Alter Anything' in a Heather Wilkinson edited book *The Perspectives of People with Dementia: Research Methods and Motivations*, published by Jessica Kingsley in 2002.

Rebecca Ley's article *Doing it for Dad* was in the Family Supplement of *The Guardian* on 8 September 2012.

Chapter Five

The quote from Danuta Lipinska comes from an article in *Pathways 10*, a newsletter produced by Dementia Services Development , University of Stirling.

Cary Smith Henderson's quote comes from *Partial View: An Alzheimer's Journal* published by Southern University Press in Dallas in 1998.

The quote from Frena Gray Davidson is from *Alzheimer's: A Practical Guide to Help You Through the Day* published by Piatkus in 1995.

Chapter Six

The anonymous quotes come from my own work.

Chapter Seven

The Will Eaves quotation is from a *Guardian* article, 'How my mother changed her mind' in the Family section.

The quote from Claire Craig appeared in a contribution titled 'Sensing Memories' in the newsletter *Pathways* which was produced by Dementia Services Development Centre, University of Stirling in 2001.

The HJ quote was in *Memories in the Making: A Program of Creative Arts Expression for Alzheimer's Patients* published by Orange County, California Alzheimer's Association in 1993.

Joan Woodward's story was in the Alzheimer's Society Newsletter in April 2001.

Stephen Davies' article was in the Alzheimer's Society Newsletter in July 1999.

Chapter Eight

Looking Into Your Voice is the title of Cathie Borrie's book published in 2010 by Nightwing Press in Vancouver, Canada.

Larry Rose's book is *Show Me the Way to go Home* and it was published by Elder Books, California in 1996.

The passage from Michael Verde is quoted from *Love, Loss and Laughter: Seeing Alzheimer's Differently* by Cathy Greenblat published in 2012 by Lyons Press, Guildford, Connecticut.

Chapter Nine

Raymond Tallis's piece comes from an article 'Manucaption' which appeared in *The Reader* 9 in 2001.

The quote from Rosemary Silcock is an extract from a play *46 Nursing Homes* broadcast on BBC Radio 4 in 1999.

The quotations from Claire Craig and Heather Hill come from personal communications.

Chapter Ten

The quotation from Beth Shirley Brough comes from her book *Alzheimer's With Love* published by Southern Cross Press in Australia in 1998.

Michael Frayn's piece is an extract from a Book Club article in *The Guardian*'s Review section on 09/06/12

Jane Crisp published *Keeping in Touch with Someone who has Alzheimer's* with Ausmed in Australia in 2000.

Chapter Eleven

The poem by Sylvia Roberts comes from the book *In the Pink* edited by myself and published by the Courtyard Centre for the Arts, Hereford in 2011.

Robert Davis's book *My Journey into Alzheimer's Disease* was published by Tyndale House: Illinois in 1989.

The Story of my Father by Susan Miller came out from Alfred A Knopf in New York in 2003.

Christine Bryden: see Chapter One.

Beverley Murphy's piece is from a contribution to the anthology *Voices of Alzheimer's* (see Chapter Eighteen).

The Creativity Press: Kansas published in 2006 Deborah Shouse's book *Love in the Land of Dementia: Finding Hope in the Caregiver's Journey.*

Chapter Twelve

Sue West's letter on 'Fiddlers' is in the Alzheimer's Society's magazine *Living with Dementia* for August 2009.

Laurel Rust's story is from 'Another Part of the Country', a contribution to *Women and Aging: An Anthology by Women* edited by Jo Alexander et al., published by Calyx Books in 1986.

The quotation from Claire Craig is from *Celebrating the Person: a Practical Approach to Arts Activities* published by Dementia Services Development Centre at the University of Stirling in 2001.

'Talking Mats' is available from the University of Stirling.

Chapter Thirteen

Frena Gray Davidson: see Chapter Five.

The extract from the article by Rosemary Clarke is from 'Precious experience beyond words' in *Journal of Dementia Care* Volume 12 No 3 in 2004.

Chapter Fourteen

Agnes Houston's remarks come from a discussion with Kate Allan and myself which was published in *Journal of Dementia Care* in 2009 (Vol 17 No 5) under the title 'The Licence to be Free: Changing the Way We See Dementia'.

Cary Smith Henderson: see Chapter Five.

Heather Hill's passage comes from *Invitation to the Dance* published by Development Dementia Centre, University of Stirling.

The Oliver Sacks quote comes from an article in the *New York Times*.

Ian McQueen's poems are to be found in my book *Dementia Diary* published by Hawker.

Chapter Fifteen

Elizabeth Cohen's *The Family at Beartown Road* was published by Harper in 2004.

Richard Taylor: see Chapter Four.

Agnes Houston: see Chapter Fourteen.

Kim Zabbia's *Painted Diaries* was published by Fairview Press, Minneapolis, USA in 1996.

Chapter Sixteen

John Zeisel's book is *I'm Still Here*. The details are under 'Further Reading'.

Laurel Rust and Amy: see Chapter Twelve.

Judith Maizel's contribution comes from *Time for Dementia* edited by Gilliard and Marshall and published by Hawker in 2010.

The anonymous quote comes from Bell and Troxel's *The Best Friends Approach to Alzheimer's Care* published by Health Communications Press.

Chapter Seventeen

The first quote is from an article 'Doing it for Dad' from the Society section of *The Guardian* for 22 September 2012.

The second is referenced under Chapter Three.

Chapter Eighteen

The first quotation comes from an article 'Hearing the Cry "I'm Still Here" in the midst of Grief and Loss' by John Zeisel, published in the *Journal of Dementia Care* Vol 18 No 2 in 2010.

All but two of the other quotations come from *Voices of Alzheimer's* edited by Betsy Peterson and published in 2004 from Da Capo Press. Debbie Booth's from *Tangles and Starbursts* edited by Bailey and Darling and published by Alzheimer's Society North Tyneside Branch in 2001.

Chapter Nineteen

This piece is based upon an article by myself and Kate Allan that appeared in *Elderly Care* Vol 11 No 1 in 1999.

Postscript

Christine Bryden: see Chapter One.

The snatches of poetry come from my books *You Are Words, Openings* and *Dementia Diary*, all published by Hawker.

The Cover photograph comes from Cathy Greenblat's book *Love, Loss and Laughter: Seeing Alzheimer's Differently* published by Lyons Press, Connecticut.

EXPLORING FURTHER

Most of the books in the field of dementia are written by specialists for specialists. They are full of medical and psychological jargon and rarely adopt a specifically positive approach. Here are two general ones, however, that could prove both helpful and inspiring:

Still Here: a Breakthrough Approach to Understanding Someone Living with Alzheimer's by John Zeisel, Piatkus: London

Love, Loss and Laughter: Seeing Alzheimer's Differently by Cathy Greenblat, Lyons Press: Connecticut

There is also a DVD which is beautiful and encouraging:

There is a Bridge made by the Memory Bridge Foundation in Chicago.

There are clips from it, and you can purchase it on www.memorybridge.org

There are other books which deal with specific aspects to which I have devoted Chapters or have referred to in them:

Counselling (Chapter Four)

Person-Centred Counselling for People with Dementia by Danuta Lipinska (Jessica Kingsley 2009)

Touch (Chapter Twelve)

Comforting Touch in Dementia and End of Life Care by Barbara Goldschmidt and Niamh van Meines (Jessica Kingsley 2011)

Creativity (Chapter Fourteen)

Creativity and Communication in Persons with Dementia by myself and Claire Craig (Jessica Kingsley 2012)

Chocolate Rain: 100 Ideas for a Creative Approach to Activities in Dementia Care by Sara Zoutewelle-Morris (Hawker 2011)

Pictures to Share books – details on www.picturestoshare.co.uk

Playfulness (Chapter Fifteen)

Playfulness and Dementia by myself (Jessica Kingsley 2013)

Living in the Moment (Chapter Sixteen)

Time for Dementia edited Gilliard and Marshall (Hawker 2010)

Remember, Remember

Hazel McHaffie

ISBN 978-1-906817-78-7 PBK £7.99

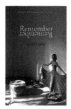

The secret has been safely kept for sixty years, but now it's on the edge of exposure.

Doris Mannering once made a choice that changed the course of her family's life. The secret was safely buried, but now with the onset of Alzheimer's her mind is wandering. She is haunted by the feeling that she must find the papers before it's too late, but she just can't remember...

Jessica is driven to despair by her mother's endless searching. But it's not until lives are in jeopardy that she consents to Doris going into a residential home. As Jessica begins clearing the family home, bittersweet memories and unexpected discoveries await her.

But these pale into insignificance against the bombshell her lawyer lover, Aaron, hands her.

Hazel McHaffie has an extraordinary ability to create the convincing inner voice of a person with severe dementia. The result is often both funny and poignant. She raises emotional and ethical issues not as theoretical 'thin' cases, but within the richly characterised world of the novel... a good read from start to finish.

PROFESSOR TONY HOPE

This moving book will resonate with anyone who has 'lost' a loved one through the living death of Alzheimer's.

SIR CLIFF RICHARD OBE

It provides an amazing insight into the thought process of someone with dementia, as well as being a gripping and heartfelt narrative.

JOURNAL OF DEMENTIA CARE

This novel, I'm sure, will resonate deeply with family members and carers trying to cope wit this most distressing condition. Recommended.

WWW.THEBOOKBAG.COM

Details of this and other books published by Luath Press can be found at: **www.luath.co.uk**

Luath Press Limited
committed to publishing well written books worth reading

LUATH PRESS takes its name from Robert Burns, whose little collie Luath (*Gael.,* swift or nimble) tripped up Jean Armour at a wedding and gave him the chance to speak to the woman who was to be his wife and the abiding love of his life. Burns called one of 'The Twa Dogs' Luath after Cuchullin's hunting dog in Ossian's *Fingal.* Luath Press was established in 1981 in the heart of Burns country, and now resides a few steps up the road from Burns' first lodgings on Edinburgh's Royal Mile.

Luath offers you distinctive writing with a hint of unexpected pleasures.

Most bookshops in the UK, the US, Canada, Australia, New Zealand and parts of Europe either carry our books in stock or can order them for you. To order direct from us, please send a £sterling cheque, postal order, international money order or your credit card details (number, address of cardholder and expiry date) to us at the address below. Please add post and packing as follows: UK – £1.00 per delivery address; overseas surface mail – £2.50 per delivery address; overseas airmail – £3.50 for the first book to each delivery address, plus £1.00 for each additional book by airmail to the same address. If your order is a gift, we will happily enclose your card or message at no extra charge.

Luath Press Limited
543/2 Castlehill
The Royal Mile
Edinburgh EH1 2ND
Scotland
Telephone: 0131 225 4326 (24 hours)
Fax: 0131 225 4324
email: sales@luath.co.uk
Website: www.luath.co.uk